WINNING THE BATTLE FOR THE BODY: A BIBLICAL STRATEGY FOR NUTRITION AND HEALTH

BY
DOUGLAS D. POLK
B.S., B.C.M., M.C.M., N.D., C.N.H.

Published by

VMI PUBLISHERS

Partnering With Christian Authors, Publishing Christian and Inspirational Books

Sisters, Oregon
www.vmipublishers.com

ISBN: 1933204192

Library of Congress Control Number: 2006922993

Author Contact:
ddpolk@alphaomegafood.com

This book is dedicated to my wife, Marilyn, and to my three children, Dale, Dean, and Daisy. Their love and support kept me on track to get this book written and published so that others could find life more abundant promised by the Lord Jesus. I am also indebted to Rev. George Malkmus, whose bold Biblical teaching on diet and lifestyle brought my wife through the most physically trying time of her life into health and vitality. Appreciation goes to Dr. Gene Fant, Department Chair & Associate Professor of English at Union University, who believed in my manuscript and encouraged me to get it published. And lastly, I owe a debt of gratitude to Dr. Adrian Rogers for his constant encouragement to me, his personal friendship, and his dynamic preaching. May his messages live on through his Love Worth Finding ministry until the Lord returns.

DISCLAIMER

"The nutritional and health information in this book is based on the teachings of God's Holy Word-the Bible, as well as personal experiences and scientific research. We do not offer medical advice or prescribe the use of diet as a form of treatment for sickness without the approval of a health professional.

Because there is always some risk involved when changing diet and lifestyles, we are not responsible for any adverse effects or consequences that might result. Please do not apply the information in this book if you are not willing to assume the risk.

If you do use the information in this book without the approval of a health professional, you are prescribing for yourself, which is your constitutional right, but Alpha Omega Food, the author, and VMI assume no responsibility."

TABLE OF CONTENTS

PREFACE
THE BATTLE FOR THE BODY

There is a battle raging between God and Satan for the physical body of every Christian. This battle is much the same as the original battle between God Almighty and the serpent, Satan, in the beautiful Garden of Eden. Adam and Eve were tempted at the very core of their humanity as their senses of sight, taste, smell, touch, and hearing were captured by a beautiful, delicious, savory, elegant FOOD that wasn't on God's allowed menu. The serpent tempted them at their greatest weakness - that which they could not live without. Our weakness has not changed. We are still very vulnerable to the temptation to let into our body that which God has said is not good for us. Has Satan changed his tactics? It doesn't seem so. Although the soul of a Christian is saved once and for all when he publicly confesses his sin and repents and asks Jesus to save him from his sin, there continues to be a war in his body between the temptations of the flesh and the discipline of the spirit-filled life.

> A mighty fortress is our God,
> A bulwark never failing;
> Our helper He amid the flood
> Of mortal ills prevailing;
> For still our ancient foe
> Doth seek to work us woe;
> His craft and pow'r are great,
> And armed with cruel hate,
> On earth is not His equal[1]

All across America, mid-week prayer meetings are one big sick-list of saints. A middle aged businessman is having a heart bypass operation, a deacon has been diagnosed with brain cancer, a neighbor has had a heart attack and that co-worker just lost a husband to lung cancer, and worst of all, children are becoming deathly sick at younger ages than ever. There is little time to pray for the lost, the broken families, the spread of the Gospel, the work of the Holy Spirit. Every person in the Sunday school class has a prayer request for some friend, family member, or themselves with various physical ailments. The body of Christ is so sick that it has to leave the front lines of battle with Satan and attend to its wounded masses. Increasing numbers of its best soldiers are falling well before their times, leaving the church without enough trained and seasoned leaders. Of course the physically sick need prayer and healing, but is it our destiny to be continually weak and sick? If we were strong and healthy, we could spend more time praying for that lost neighbor, that Christian Senator, that lost judge, the schools and teachers, and the missionaries on the front lines all across the world. Corporate prayer has been taken over by a drudgery of diseases. Some Christians avoid prayer meetings altogether because they see them as futile and ineffectual. Have we come to the point where we only have time to pray for healing of the physically sick, or for those who have lost loved ones to illness?

Next time there's a gathering of ministers, take a look at us. Most ministers are overweight, others are obese, and more than a few are very obese. It's no wonder that ministers are among the most expensive to insure. Not only are we under great pressure of the ministry, but we are also some of the most unhealthy people on earth.

It's no wonder. What do we do at most church gatherings? Feasting and playing have taken the place of fasting and praying! The most dangerous foods are often the buffets laid out at our church socials. Pot lucks have led to pot guts. You'll likely see more healthy food at a steak house than at the church banquet! Casseroles, cakes, fried chicken, roast beef, ham, barbequed pork, pizza, pastries, and breads grace the tables along with plenty of sweet tea, and of course, diet sodas. Youth gatherings commonly lavish pizzas, chicken, hot dogs, hamburgers, greasy chips, and a hefty supply of sugary soft drinks. Standard Sunday school morning treats are doughnuts, sausage biscuits, coffee, pasteurized orange juice, and soft drinks. Rarely do you find raw fruits and vegetables, green salads, pure water, and other healthy fare. Even though the Center for Disease Control says that we have an epidemic of diabetes, the church barrels on with abandon toward supplying every sweet available to our worshipers.

Heard any sermons on gluttony lately? Probably not. It can be suicide for a minister to attack the very basic appetites of mankind, especially if he himself is no model of temperance. Is it politically correct to pray for the alcoholic to get control of his addiction and so politically incorrect to pray for the glutton to get control of his appetite? For the same reason that there is no "Chocoholics Anonymous" there are no rules of overindulgence when it comes to eating. No one wants to quit! No one wants to be told what to eat and what not to eat. It's the same old sin that got mankind into trouble from the start.

> And the LORD God commanded the man, saying, Of every tree of the garden thou mayest freely eat: But of the tree of the knowledge of good and evil, thou shalt not eat of it: for in the day that thou eatest thereof thou shalt surely die.[2]

When Adam and Eve decided to be their own boss, it was pertaining to food, and then came our downfall. Satan, the master tempter and liar, appealed to their physical cravings and told them that they would not die if they ate the fruit. They disobeyed God and they became separated from their Holy Creator because of their selfish desires.

The flesh is so closely tied to the spirit that if we are disobedient in one, then we are disobedient in the other also. If we refuse physical discipline, we also refuse spiritual discipline. As you shall see later in this book, this fact was also demonstrated in the wilderness experience of God's people, the Israelites, when escaping slavery from Egypt. At the core of holiness is the discipline of spirit, soul and body.

Christians have been taught that the first sin was a general sin of trying to be our own god. Be that as it may, we have neglected the fact that it was a specific sin, gluttony, that brought our downfall. Gluttony, as defined in Webster's Dictionary is:

1 : excess in eating or drinking
2 : greedy or excessive indulgence[3]

Because Adam and Eve did not want to abide by God's boundaries of what to eat and drink, they suffered and as a general consequence, we have suffered. Lack of boundaries in eating and drinking has caused mankind literally to fall from life and health. And we have neglected that specific sin throughout history and denied that we have a problem of fleshly lust for food and drink. We have repeatedly chosen the wrong foods and beverages and it has led us into disease and brevity of life.

Many Christians equate freedom from the consequences of sin to mean freedom from the discipline of restraint in food and beverages. Time after time godly men and women are taken from us in the prime of their lives by heart attacks, cancer, and stroke. Time after time great servants of the Lord are relegated to hospitals, rest homes, and sick beds because of disease. There is much work to be done, but God's people are stuck in the mire of physical or mental sickness brought on by gluttony. Christians are eating the same foods as the heathen. We have taken the scripture in Acts too literally and substituted license for liberty.

> And there came a voice to him, Rise, Peter; kill, and eat. But Peter said, Not so, Lord; for I have never eaten any thing that is common or unclean.[4]

God has not cleansed meat of its dangerous animal fat and cholesterol, its animal protein that stresses the liver and kidneys, nor the chemical additives and infectious diseases that it now carries. Just as He has allowed divorce and the eating of animal flesh, it is not His original plan, because it is not His perfect will, but His permissive will. The true meaning of this passage is explained by Peter later in verse 34 and 35.

> Then Peter opened *his* mouth, and said, Of a truth I perceive that God is no respecter of persons: But in every nation he that feareth him, and worketh righteousness, is accepted with him.[5]

Here Peter realized that God was showing him that the Gospel is for all mankind, not that dangerous foods were now permitted. Peter says that those who revere the Lord and are obedient to His laws are welcomed into His kingdom regardless of their nationality or station in life. When taken too literally, we can use this verse as a license to eat and drink without regard to God's original menu for health. This passage has been misunderstood at the peril of our physical lives.

Christians are supposed to be temples of the Holy Spirit of Jesus Christ, God Almighty. The temple of God should be holy, pure, strong, beautiful, well-built, well-kept, and full of life. But most of us Christians are unsightly, weak, overweight, out of shape, and suffering from degenerative diseases that are caused by an undisciplined diet and lifestyle.

Of course, Christians are like everyone else in that they want good health; it's just that they aren't ready to pay the price to achieve it. George Barna's research states:

> "Of 21 possible goals for the future, adults rated good health as their most coveted future reality - by a considerable margin. Nine out of ten adults cherish good physical health. That outcome was the top-rated goal of Americans a decade ago, too." [6]

Sure, we want health, but do we really want to pay the price for it? **Actual causes of death** contribute to this nation's leading killers including heart disease, cancer, and stroke. The U. S. Center for Disease Control defines Actual Cause of Death as **lifestyle and behavioral**. In 2000, the most common actual causes of death in the United States were tobacco (435,000), poor diet and physical inactivity (400,000), alcohol consumption (85,000), microbial agents (e.g., influenza and pneumonia, 75,000), toxic agents (e.g., pollutants and asbestos, 55,000), motor vehicle accidents (43,000), firearms (29,000), sexual behavior (20,000) and illicit use of drugs (17,000).

> Dallas, TX — June 18, 2003 — During the Annuity Board report to the Southern Baptist Convention, President O.S. Hawkins challenged pastors and church staff members to "take care of yourself physically and treat your body as the temple of the Holy Spirit. If our people began to take responsibility for their health and adopt an attitude of wellness, we would see insurance claims and monthly payments decline," Hawkins said. [7]

Could you pick out the Christians in a lineup of a cross section of people from all walks of life? No. Christians are just like the rest of the world. Shouldn't Christians be different in appearance as well as conduct? Shouldn't we stick out in a crowd? Of course there would still be short and tall - but would there be obese and very obese Christians? What if the rest of the world could look at us and say "I've noticed that you are never sick, and you are so trim and strong! How do you do it?" What if the rest of the world could see us as healthy and full of vitality? Wouldn't they want the message of the gospel even more? Wouldn't' they be more likely to believe it? Daniel and his friends stuck out because they took care of their body temples and wouldn't eat the king's food.

> Then said Daniel to Melzar, whom the prince of the eunuchs had set over Daniel, Hananiah, Mishael, and Azariah, Prove thy servants, I beseech thee, ten days; and let them give us pulse[vegetables] to eat, and water to drink. Then let our countenances be looked upon before thee, and the countenance of the children that eat of the portion of the king's meat: and as thou seest, deal with thy servants. So he consented to them in this matter, and proved them ten days. And at the end of ten days their countenances appeared fairer and fatter in flesh than all the children which did eat the portion of the king's meat.[8]

I believe that God wants His church to be the spotless bride, in love with Jesus and telling the whole world of her upcoming marriage to the Lamb. I believe it's time to renovate our temples and remodel our tabernacles by rethinking our diets and lifestyles. It's time to get healthy and be about the work of telling a sick world that only Jesus saves soul, spirit, AND body! This book will seek to convince you, the reader, that you and I and all Christians need to renovate our body temples by leaving behind the world's false foods, return to God's original diet, and worship Him with all of our soul, with all of our spirit, and with all of our body.

> And the very God of peace sanctify you wholly; and *I pray God* your whole spirit and soul and body be preserved blameless unto the coming of our Lord Jesus Christ.[9]

---

[1] *Logos Hymnal*. 1st edition. Oak Harbor, WA: Logos Research Systems, Inc., 1995.

[2] *The Holy Bible : King James Version.*, Ge 2:16-17. Oak Harbor, WA: Logos Research Systems, Inc., 1995.

[3] Merriam-Webster, Inc. *Merriam-Webster's Collegiate Dictionary*. Includes Index. 10th ed. Springfield, Mass., U.S.A.: Merriam-Webster, 1996, c1993.

[4] *The Holy Bible : King James Version.*, Ac 10:13-14. Oak Harbor, WA: Logos Research Systems, Inc., 1995.

[5]*The Holy Bible : King James Version.*, Ac 10:34-35. Oak Harbor, WA: Logos Research Systems, Inc., 1995.

[6]Barna, George. Americans Identify What They Want Out of Life, April 26, 2000 *The Barna Update* (September 2, 2005). *http://www.barna.org/FlexPage.aspx?Page=BarnaUpdate&BarnaUpdateID=57*

[7]O.S. Hawkins, *Exec Challenges Pastors to Take Responsibility for Their Health*, Wednesday, Jun 18, 2003, By Jerilynn Armstrong, Phoenix (Baptist Press)

[8]*The Holy Bible : King James Version.*, Da 1:11-15. Oak Harbor, WA: Logos Research Systems, Inc., 1995.

[9]*The Holy Bible : King James Version.*, 1 Th 5:23. Oak Harbor, WA: Logos Research Systems, Inc., 1995.

PROLOGUE: IN THE BEGINNING

(According to the inspired Word of God, and various creation science models, this is a probable scenario of what life was like in the beginning.)

Lets' journey back to the beginning of time - back to the perfect world that God created in just six days by simply speaking it into existence. Imagine the universe in the beginning. God created it completely perfect and perfectly mature. The planets, the stars, the earth are mathematically in sync with one another. No errant meteors are flying through space and hitting planets and stars. All things are in harmony with God and with each other.

You are there with Adam and Eve with all the finest food anyone could want just waiting to be picked and eaten. Thousands of varieties of fruits and vegetables, nuts and seeds abound in the Garden of Eden. You wake up in the morning refreshed by the night's sleep on a bed of lush grass. Eight feet tall, with little fat on your lean, naked body you stretch as the night is slowly being washed away. A gentle, diffused light comes from the sun as it peeks through the beautiful blue water canopy that completely covers the earth miles up in the atmosphere.

The air is abundantly rich in oxygen, giving you bounding energy in every breath, and carbon dioxide provides fuel for plants to manufacture food. The ground is saturated with water from below and a mist arises in the morning and waters the insects and animals at the beginning of each new day. There are no clouds in the sky - but don't worry, the sun won't burn you because the canopy shields the earth from its destructive radiation. Because the earth's axis is always vertical, there is only one season and that season is a marvelous growing period of endless duration. Night is gently transformed into day as the canopy disperses the light gradually over the terminator.

The most unusual thing about this garden is that no creature feeds on another creature. There is no killing, no eating of one species by another, for God has created the plants to feed the animals and the plants are fed in turn by the rich, moist, dirt, glorious sunlight, and the abundant carbon dioxide atmosphere.

Each plant is created with its own special coloring, its unique nutritional spectrum, and its distinctive taste to fulfill a particular requirement of each of God's creatures. One plant provides leaves that are especially satisfying, while another yields crunchy nuts or delicious fruits. Programmed into you by your Maker, you and the animals instinctively seek out certain roots and herbs for a particular dietary need. An unnumbered variety of seeds and grains supply a cereal menu second to none. Myriad varieties of flowers, grasses, and trees, parade by you as you drink in the visual and aromatic variety before you daily.

The streams and lakes are teeming with colorful aquatic life. The humidity, temperature, and atmospheric pressure are in such balance that there has never been any rain. You relax under your daily shower at one of dozens of waterfalls. God communes with you as you spend your day enjoying Him and His creation.

There is no killing, no death, and no sickness in this truly utopian kingdom. Every species is free of disease or infestation by any other specie. Viruses and bacteria have not mutated into the deadly microbes they became after the Fall. There are animals of all sizes living free and peaceable together with you in God's perfect garden. The so-called food chain of modern science does not exist. The zoological world is totally dependent upon the botanical world. This scenario is not far fetched. It is within the very possible and probable. Many scientists who are Christian believe that such a wonderful world actually did exist.

> And God said, Behold, I have given you every herb bearing seed, which *is* upon the face of all the earth, and every tree, in the which *is* the fruit of a tree yielding seed; to you it shall be for meat. And to every beast of the earth, and to every fowl of the air, and to every thing that creepeth upon the earth, wherein *there is* life, *I have given* every green herb for meat: and it was so.[1]

This book is different. We will take a different attitude and a different viewpoint than most of the other interpreters of the Biblical revelation as to the body, its health and well-being. We will try to glean from the Holy Scripture a healthy view of the real battle that is going on for the physical body of mankind. So get ready for a fresh look at the Lord's plan for abundant life promised to us by God but short-circuited by the devil's crafty plan of temptation and destruction.

After having read these truths it is my prayer that you will be in agreement that you don't have to be sick because sickness is not normal. I pray that you can come to the realization that we can go back to the Garden lifestyle and return to the health and wellness that God intended for us to enjoy.

> Encamped along the hills of light,
> Ye Christian soldiers, rise,
> And press the battle ere the night
> Shall veil the glowing skies.
> Against the foe in vales below,
> Let all our strength be hurled;
> Faith is the victory, we know,
> That overcomes the world.[2]

---

[1] *The Holy Bible : King James Version., Ge 1:29-30. Oak Harbor, WA: Logos Research Systems, Inc., 1995.*
[2] *Faith Is the Victory, John Yates.*

CHAPTER 1

BATTLE PLAN A

The Master's Menu: First Fast Foods

The devil knew that man was free to choose his own course, so he capitalized on the desire in man to make his own decisions and to disregard God's way.

> And when the woman saw that the tree *was* good for food, and that it *was* pleasant to the eyes, and a tree to be desired to make *one* wise, she took of the fruit thereof, and did eat, and gave also unto her husband with her; and he did eat.[1]

In the Garden of Eden, Adam and Eve had the best of all possible worlds. Twenty-first century fast foods are no match for the original fast foods that the Creator provided. Having it our way has led the world into disease and death. Recently, a rash of law suits against America's fast food giants has drawn attention to the dangers of fast food menus. A news release from the Physicians Committee for Responsible Medicine dated July, 2002 said:

> "This is no doubt just the first of many lawsuits holding the food industry at least partially to blame for America's diet-related epidemics," says PCRM president and nutrition researcher Neal D. Barnard, M.D. "Decades of scientific evidence show that the cholesterol and saturated fat in beef, chicken, pork, and dairy products dramatically increase the risk of colon cancer, diabetes, heart disease, stroke, obesity, and other diseases." [2]

HAVE IT HIS WAY

God is the perfect Chef. He is the Master Nutritionist and Dietician of dieticians. He is every doctor's Doctor. He is the PhD's PhD. There is no one who is His equal in formulating a diet for health. There is no better fast food than His fast food. His is packaged perfectly and you can even eat the package and not litter the countryside with paper and Styrofoam! So why go to anyone else for the best food and the best diet? Just think about it. Each food has its own beautiful color and shape, texture and mixture of taste-tantalizing ingredients. Just the sight of natural foods starts the digestive juices flowing.

In the Garden, the trees and plants were constantly loaded with ripe fruit just asking to be picked and eaten by Adam, Eve, and the animals. Only in the past two hundred years have we discovered the variety of nutrients that are available in raw fruits, raw vegetables, raw nuts, and raw seeds.

> I sing the goodness of the Lord,
> That filled the earth with food;
> He formed the creatures with His Word,
> And then pronounced them good.[3]

THE PERFECT DIET

It is a scientific fact that life begets life (biogenesis). It's the same with food. Live food begets life. Dead food begets death. In God's original plan, mankind and the animals were to eat live food - food filled with life. What is live food? All live foods have three common characteristics necessary for the health of our bodies.

God's foods were intended to be eaten **raw**, insuring the full spectrum of phytochemicals, vitamins, micro-minerals, and enzymes that He built into each one to enable proper assimilation by the body. Heat (above 118 degrees Fahrenheit) inactivates some of the natural enzymes in the raw food. If these enzymes are destroyed by heat, light, radiation, or oxidation, the body is missing some of the synergy of combined nutrients. Although there is little scientific evidence that the enzymes in raw food aid in digestion, the cooked food is definitely missing some nutritional value, even though some nutrients in cooked foods may be absorbed better by cooking.

God's foods were intended to be eaten **fresh**. Even though God packaged our food ingeniously, as soon as the fruit, vegetable, nut, or seed is removed from the vital life support of the stem, root, limb, or vine, it begins to deteriorate and spoil. Fresh, raw food has maximum nutrition. Raw foods, except for seeds and nuts, have very short shelf lives.

God's food must be unchanged, unbroken, and **pure**, without any additional additives found in today's highly-processed foods. These additives are fractured nutrients that the body must complete before they can be assimilated as food. Additives are also treated as toxins by the body and must be eliminated or stored. Seeds that have been genetically-altered have consequences that we can only guess. Food that has been microwaved has been subjected to extreme molecular bombardment, creating a great amount of heat and possibly destroying nutrients.

Therefore, the three criteria for healthful foods are that they must be raw, fresh, and unaltered by mankind. These criteria result in foods that supply complete nutrients that do not require additional input by the body in order to make them assimilatable, nor do they require detoxification to render them harmless. They do not contain unbalanced nutritional ingredients, which can destroy the acid-alkaline balance necessary for proper pH.

God made the world perfect. The diet He gave us was expressly made for mankind and the animals. Contemporary diets that are most effective in bringing health are the ones most like the Genesis 1:29 diet. Joel Robbins, M.D., N.D, D.C, a leader in promoting the natural lifestyle who operates a very successful Wellness Clinic in Tulsa, Oklahoma, states,

> "Our bodies are designed to live and operate in health on one type of fuel only: raw fruits and vegetables, nuts, and whole grains."[4]

Joel Fuhrman, M.D, has attracted much attention with his medical practice in New Jersey in which he uses natural rather than medicinal methods to treat his patients. A former Olympic figure skating champion, Dr. Fuhrman is the author of such books as Fasting and Eating for Health, Eat to Live, and Disease-Proof Your Child. Dr. Fuhrman gives this observation about plant foods.

"Many studies show that raw fruits and vegetables offer the highest blood levels of cancer-protective nutrients and the most protection against cancer of any other foods, including cooked vegetation. Any advice not recognizing that raw vegetables and fresh fruits are the two most powerful anti-cancer categories of foods is off the mark."[5]

The Physicians Committee for Responsible Medicine, a national organization of medical doctors who advocate preventative health care, suggest a low-fat, and low-cholesterol diet that moves away from meat and dairy products. The PCRM recently released information on the health effects of the most popular diets. Only two of the 11 top-selling books got PCRM's top rating: Eat More, Weigh Less, by Dean Ornish, MD, and The McDougall Program for Maximum Weight Loss, by John McDougall, MD. Both promote low-fat vegetarian diets, high in fiber, and low in cholesterol.

So why is God's original diet perfect? Because He, the Great Physician, created it. From what we can determine, it is exactly what the body requires for life and health. Let's look at the requirements of the body for proper nutrition. Most nutritionists agree that the body needs the macronutrients called carbohydrates, fats, and protein for life, as well as fiber for cleansing of wastes. An increasing number of health professionals also say that raw foods including raw fruits, raw vegetables, raw nuts, and raw seeds, contain all the necessary macronutrients as well as the micronutrients such as vitamins, minerals, phytochemicals, enzymes, and fiber vital for life, which cannot be duplicated in processed foods or synthetic supplements.

The new food pyramids released by the USDA in mid-2005 demonstrate that a plant based diet is sufficient for providing total nutrition.

Protein has many important functions in the body and is essential for growth and maintenance. Protein needs can easily be met by eating a variety of plant-based foods. Combining different protein sources in the same meal is not necessary. Sources of protein for vegetarians include beans, nuts, nut butters, peas, and soy products (tofu, tempeh, veggie burgers).[6]

Rev. George Malkmus, author of <u>God's Way to Ultimate Health</u>, and founder of Hallelujah Acres lifestyle center, says:

> "My personal conviction after almost 20 years of research is that if we could get people off the animal products (meat and dairy), sugar, salt, white flour products and drugs, and onto a new diet with lots of raw vegetable juices...that not only could we eliminate the causes of almost all sickness from the world, but we could restore emotional and mental health to most people." [7]

The largest nutritional study ever conducted found conclusive evidence that a plant-based diet avoids the degenerative diseases that beset most Americans. T. Colin Campbell, PhD., writing in the book, <u>The China Project</u>, reveals the fantastic findings of this monumental study.

> "The China-Oxford-Cornell Project, begun in 1983 is a collaborative effort between Cornell University, the Chinese Academy of Preventive Medicine, the Chinese Academy of Medical Sciences, and Oxford University, England, as well as scientists from the United States, China, Britain, France, and other countries. China was chosen for this study because it is a living laboratory. This is because the Chinese, unlike our restless population, tend to spend their entire lives in the same area and eat the same kinds of locally-grown foods throughout their lives. Diets in China vary considerably from one region to another, so one can study the effect of diet on health like no other study has ever done. This study is the most comprehensive database on the multiple causes of disease ever compiled. In 1983 and again in 1989, American, Chinese, and English researchers gathered information on how people live and die in 65 counties in various parts of China. This study showed conclusively that only small intakes of animal products were associated with significant increases in chronic degenerative diseases." [8]

Battle Plan A has been rediscovered in our time. We have uncovered evidence after evidence that the Lord's first diet was and still is the best diet for mankind in the battle for the body.

THE REAL FOOD CHAIN

Scientists in our day have invented a name for the cycle of predation that has arisen after the fall of man. It's called the food chain and it simply orders the eating of plants by animals and animals by animals. However, God's original design was for mankind and the animal kingdom to eat only plants. Ken Ham, in his book, The Lie, Evolution, says

> "Man and animals were created to be vegetarian. This, of course, fits with the fact that there was no death before Adam's fall. But because of the entrance of sin into the world, death resulted. Sin affected the world so much that God caused a flood to come upon the earth in judgment. Genesis 6:12-13 (KJV) states: *"And God looked upon the earth, and behold it was corrupt; for all flesh had corrupted his way upon the earth. And God said unto Noah, The end of all flesh is come before me; for the earth is filled with violence through them; and, behold, I will destroy them with the earth.* Part of this violence could have been the animals starting to kill each other and perhaps man, and vice versa. Actually, though, man was not given specific instructions from God that he could eat meat until after Noah's Flood." [9]

The Institute for Creation Research points out that the original plan of God in the Bible was for the animals to be totally sustained by the plant kingdom. In spite of the evolutionist claim that some animals were designed to be carnivorous (meat eaters), **the Bible clearly indicates that they were all designed to be herbivorous.**

> Neither man nor the animals were intended originally to be carnivorous, but to eat fruits and herbs only. It is possible, even today, for both man and the carnivorous animals to survive on vegetarian diets if they have to. Furthermore, neither man nor animals were originally intended to die, possessing as they do the nephesh, or "soul," or "creature," the principle of conscious life that plants do not possess (Genesis 1:21, 24; 2:7). [10]

PLANT-FED ANIMALS

Why have we so disregarded the Biblical record in Genesis about plant-based food? And why did God institute this menu for us? Why are plants good for us? Let's investigate this for a moment.

In order for the human body to thrive, it must have live food. Live food is food that contains carbohydrates, fats, and proteins, as well as the micronutrients that comprise the absolutely vital needs of the body. Live food also contains cellulose or fiber that is needed to carry waste out of our body. Ingeniously included into these necessary ingredients are enzymes and phytochemicals that are the life force of the foods. God designed plants to provide that supply of necessary nutrients and liveness. Only plants have a design that allows the chemical process of photosynthesis to provide food for animals.

carbon dioxide ..water....sunlight....in the presence of chlorophyll...yields sugar...and oxygen

$$6\ CO_2 + 6\ H_2O + \text{Radiant Energy} \longrightarrow C_6H_{12}O_6 + 6O_2$$

Photosynthesis changes inorganic minerals from the dirt into organic compounds that can be assimilated by animals and mankind. Animals and mankind cannot perform photosynthesis and thus cannot provide the entire spectrum of foods that man and the animal kingdom demand for life. Even so-called carnivorous animals must eat herbivorous animals in order to survive and they must eat them raw, with the enzymes and phytochemicals intact.

The three types of enzymes are metabolic, digestive, and food enzymes. Metabolic enzymes are present everywhere in the body and act as catalysts for virtually every action of the body. Digestive enzymes are manufactured by the body for the purpose of breaking down food particles allowing the assimilation of the foods we eat. Food enzymes are contained in the live food we eat and these enzymes can improve immune function and have other nutritional value to humans that scientists are just beginning to discover..

Why not eat all our food cooked? Well, only the raw food retains all those delicate food factors that are so fragile and life-giving. The enzymes in plants are very sensitive to heat, light, chemicals, and radiation. If the temperature rises above 107 degrees Fahrenheit, the enzymes begin to die and at 122 degrees Fahrenheit almost all are inactivated or chemically modified.

In a biochemical sense, enzymes are proteins that can be denatured, or made ineffectual, as the dictionary explains:

> **de·na·ture** *Biochemistry.*
> To cause the tertiary structure of (a protein) to unfold, as with heat, alkali, or acid, so that some of its original properties, especially its biological activity, are diminished or eliminated.[11]

A vivid example of how important enzymes are to life is the all-too-common story of how the lady left her child in a hot car as she went into the grocery store. The child, after having been exposed to heat in excess of 120 degrees Fahrenheit for only a few minutes, is irreversibly dead because the body temperature has reached levels above 107 degrees Fahrenheit. When enzymes die or are denatured, all metabolism stops and death ensues.

The same effect can be seen in a carrot which is fresh and stiff. Boil it or heat it in an oven for a few minutes and it becomes limp. Such a carrot will not re-sprout because it is dead. If we eat food that is cooked at temperatures above 122 degrees, we are eating dead food. That means that the body will be missing the enzymes, some vitamins, and who knows how many phytochemicals that are denatured by the high heat. Also the fiber that was firm and strong is weakened by the cooking action, and is less a broom for cleaning the colon. In fact, most of the food Americans eat today is worse than just cooked; it is highly processed and contains not even a fragment of the symphony of nutrients that God intended for us to receive if we ate the foods growing on the earth.

Another reason for eating raw plants is that there is a great need for the body to have an alkaline pH rather than an acid pH. Your blood must have a pH of 7.4 in order for you to live. If your blood pH varies from that just a tenth of a point, you are in trouble, and if it varies two tenths of a point, you are dead. Only raw plants have an alkaline pH that our body needs. When we eat animal flesh, we don't get any alkalinity, only acidity. Even uncooked acid fruits appear to digest and leave an alkaline ash in our digestive tract. Cooked animal flesh leaves an acid residue that must be neutralized by our body's innately intelligent cells. What mineral source do our cells have for neutralizing acidity? The calcium in our bones and our teeth are the only adequate source for neutralization of acid ash and this could be one of the reasons that we are one of the leading nations in osteoporosis, or porous bones.

The plant-based diet satisfies the original programmed operation of metabolism in our body. The cells of our body have what is called "innate intelligence". God programmed into every cell through DNA coding an algorithm of orders and plans to equip it for health. Our cells only know how to stay healthy. They will go to any length to guard the body from invaders such as toxins, synthetics, foreign matter, or anything else that is not natural to the health of the body. Only recently have we been able to overcome this innate intelligence with drugs which turn off the immune system and make heart, lung, and other organ transplants possible.

FORBIDDEN FRUIT: ENDLESS ERROR

In the Garden of Eden God commanded that Adam and Eve not eat of the tree of the knowledge of good and evil. Of course there are spiritual implications of this command, but I believe that there are physical ones as well. Granted, God knows what is harmful to us and what is healthful. Man was and is ignorant of what is in our best interests. Only our Creator is omniscient, omnipresent, and omnipotent. He knew that for us to have the knowledge of good and evil was for us to also have the potential for sin. The scripture in James 4:11-17 says *"Therefore to him that knoweth to do good, and doeth it not, to him it is sin."* It should be obvious to the reader that there was something in that forbidden fruit that was not good for mankind. God knew it and man didn't know it or did not believe it. That's still our problem today. We think that we know more than God about food and about life. We become our own gods. We sin.

So what happened? Why is the world so different? Because of sin. Because of sin we no longer have perfect water, perfect atmosphere, perfect food, or perfect companionship. And what was the first sin? Disobedience to God in what to eat.

And unto Adam he said, Because thou hast hearkened unto the voice of thy wife, and hast eaten of the tree, of which I commanded thee, saying, Thou shalt not eat of it: cursed *is* the ground for thy sake; in sorrow shalt thou eat *of* it all the days of thy life; Thorns also and thistles shall it bring forth to thee; and thou shalt eat the herb of the field; In the sweat of thy face shalt thou eat bread, till thou return unto the ground; for out of it wast thou taken: for dust thou *art*, and unto dust shalt thou return.[12]

 Because of sin, man can no longer live in a perfect place and he must eventually die physically. God expelled us from that perfect place and now we have to live in a cursed world – a world where killing is second nature, or more accurately, natural. Naturally we kill other animals to eat. Naturally animals kill other animals for food. Naturally species feed on other species, kinds feed on other kinds, and even some plants, such as the Venus Fly Trap, feed on animals.

---

[1] *The Holy Bible : King James Version.*, Genesis 3:6. Oak Harbor, WA: Logos Research Systems, Inc., 1995.

[2] Barnard, Neal. http://www.pcrm.org/news/health020726.html.

[3] I Sing the Mighty Power of God, Isaac Watts.

[4] Robbins, Joel. Juicing for Health. R.W. Graybill & Company, Tulsa, OK. 2001. pg.9

[5] Furhman, Joel. Eat to Live. Little, Brown, and Company Boston, New York, London. 2003. pg.43

[6] Vegetarian Diets, MyPyramid.gov, United States Department of Agriculture, http://www.mypyramid.gov/tips_resources/vegetarian_diets.html, Aug. 23, 2005.

[7] Malkmus, George. God's Way to Ultimate Health. p.75

[8] Campbell, T. Colin and Cox, Christine. The China Project. New Century Nutrition, 1996.

[9] Ham, Keith. The Lie, Evolution Creation-Life Publishers, El Cajon, CA, p.142.

[10] http://www.icr.org/bible/bhta46.html

[11] http://dictionary.reference.com/search?q=denatured

[12] *The Holy Bible : King James Version.*, Genesis 3:17-19. Oak Harbor, WA: Logos Research Systems, Inc., 1995.

CHAPTER 2

FALL FROM FRUIT-FULL-NESS

The First Sacrifice

Original sin had a tremendous cost. Because Adam and Eve disobeyed God, there was a debt to be paid that could only be paid by the shedding of blood. Because God is holy and just, sin must be punished. Instead of killing Adam and Eve, our loving God had to kill an animal and make clothing for them because they realized that they were naked. A sacrifice had to be made because of sin. Of course, the killing of the animal did not wipe away man's sin, but it provided a picture of the problem and the solution that would eventually come one day. The clothing God provided Adam and Eve by the death of an animal provided protection for them and a covering for the nakedness that their sin had exposed. This is the picture of what Jesus did for us on the cross. He provided a covering for our sin by His death on that cross.

> Blessed *is he whose* transgression *is* forgiven, *whose* sin *is* covered.[1]

> For since by man *came* death, by man *came* also the resurrection of the dead.[2]

Mankind, Adam and Eve, committed the first sin by their disobedience to God. The punishment for sin is and has always been death. The forgiveness for sin has always been at the price of shed blood. But God chose to require the death of an animal instead of the death of the man or woman. That may seem the easy way out to some, but I believe that it grieved God to have to kill an animal, especially the perfect animals that He had just made. This did not pay for their sin, because it was not a high enough sacrifice. It took the price of precious blood of the Lord Jesus Christ to pay mankind's sin debt. **However, as we shall see, God kept reminding them of the high price of sin by demanding that they sacrifice the very finest, first fruits of their flocks and herds each and every time they sinned.**

THE CURSE

So Satan and the ground were cursed by God, and animal life was sacrificed to show mankind the error of sin. Death entered into the perfect world that God had made. Man's appetite for forbidden fruit began the struggle for survival in a vastly different world. Adam and Eve were not given a "free ride" anymore. The door to the Garden of Eden was shut tight and they were cast out into a world that was changed in a moment from a sacred place to a scary place.

> And the LORD God said, Behold, the man is become as one of us, to know good and evil: and now, lest he put forth his hand, and take also of the tree of life, and eat, and live for ever: Therefore the LORD God sent him forth from the garden of Eden, to till the ground from whence he was taken. So he drove out the man; and he placed at the east of the garden of Eden Cherubims, and a flaming sword which turned every way, to keep the way of the tree of life.[3]

EVICTION FROM EDEN

This began a very different way of life for mankind. Some dynamic changes occurred. **Killing entered the world and the animal kingdom began to feed on itself.** We have very little information on whether disease entered the world at that time, but we know that killing became a part of life. Adam and Eve's firstborn, Cain became a farmer and his brother Abel became a sheep herder. Cain's offering to the Lord was of the fruit of the ground that had been cursed. Abel's offering to the Lord was from the blood of an animal that he had to kill. Cain became jealous of his brother's favor with God so he killed Abel.

God not only locked mankind away from the Tree of Life, but also took away perfect food, although we can only guess to what extent. Adam and Eve and all their descendents would have to work for their food by planting, fertilizing, watering, guarding, and harvesting it, saving some seeds to plant again. Unlike the unimpeded lush growth in the Garden, there were weeds, thorns, thistles, briars and probably ravaging insects and harmful microbes in this cursed, cruel world.

As a result of the curse of the ground, Adam and Eve and the rest of us were forced to eat not only limited amounts of the remaining fruits, but also the plants of the field, herbs. That is, we had to eat grass, leaves, stems, blossoms, roots, and such since fruit was in very limited supply. We can live on these herbs but they are not as densely nutritious and as easily digested as fruits.

Sweat for Sweets

The first mention of bread in the Biblical record comes here in Genesis 3:19. Bread is a processed food. It can only be made by taking mature grain and processing it by grinding it into flour, and mixing it with leaven, oil, and water to make dough. Then the dough is heated and the leavening causes it to rise until it becomes bread. Grain became a food that could be stored, then processed and eaten. Grain is not a real food. It is very limited in nutrition because it has to be cooked, killing live enzymes and destroying some vitamins and minerals. It is also an acid food that works against the body's natural alkaline pH. But whole grain does provide starch and glucose for energy and some fiber if the bran is still intact. Throughout the remainder of history, cereal grains have provided a sustainable, yet imperfect food supply for mankind and the animals.

Today in America, breads and cereals are touted by the United States Department of Agriculture as the base food in their so-called "food pyramid". While this suggested diet pyramid, first published in 1992, contains the original fruits and vegetables, it also includes animal products. The new pyramids, which were published in April, 2005 still include meats and dairy since political and financial pressure groups

exert tremendous influence on the USDA. There is very little
nutritionally-sound science reflected in the food pyramids. The food
pyramid for best health is still the one from Genesis 1:29-30 in which
fruits and vegetables are the primary need for mankind with limited nuts
and seeds and no animal or processed foods (see Hallelujah Diet
Pyramid, pg.135).

God made physical death a certainty when He expelled man from
the Garden. Why? Because the new diet outside the Garden was one
that would lead to death. Killing had entered the perfect world so that
the animal kingdom would eventually kill itself.

LONGEVITY AGAINST DEPRAVITY

The new diet without perfect fruit and vegetables was certain to
bring physical death eventually. But the world was still a pretty good
place to live compared to today. There was still a water canopy and a
dense atmosphere of oxygen in this cursed world. Even though the
ground was cursed there were still giant animals and giant men.
Disease was very rare, if present at all. The fossil record shows that
there were giant animals (dinosaurs), giant plants (sequoias), and giant
men. The Bible called these giant men Nephilim (Gen. 6:4 and Num.
13:33), who were over nine feet tall.

Most of the world was still land and rainfall had not yet come upon
the earth. The vegetation that remained was prevalent over the entire
world, yet not as perfect as in the Garden. The Bible tells us in the fifth
chapter of Genesis that even after the Fall, mankind lived a very long
time and then died. These men lived to an average of over 900 years of
age and produced many offspring. There is no record in the Bible that
men ate the animals for food during this time. There was so much food
in abundance that there obviously was no need to eat animal flesh. And
God had not yet given men permission to kill the animals for food.

According to New Nave's Topical Bible, the ages of the pre-flood
men of Genesis were as follows: Adam lived 930 years, Seth lived 912
years, Enos lived 905 years, Cainan lived 910 years, Mahalaleel lived
895 years, Jared lived 962 years, Enoch lived 365 years (and didn't die
but was taken away by God), Methuselah lived 969 years (the record),

Lamech lived 777 years, and Noah lived 950 years. All these men died
except Enoch, who according to Genesis 5:23 did not die. [4]

> And all the days of Enoch were three hundred sixty and five
> years: And Enoch walked with God: and he *was* not; for God
> took him. [5]

In the days that followed, mankind became more and more
corrupted. The longevity and depravity of the people got them into more
and more trouble. God lost His patience and finally decided to limit the
lifespan of His crowning creation.

> And it came to pass, when men began to multiply on the face
> of the earth, and daughters were born unto them, That the
> sons of God saw the daughters of men that they *were* fair; and
> they took them wives of all which they chose. And the LORD
> said, My spirit shall not always strive with man, for that he
> also *is* flesh: yet his days shall be an hundred and twenty
> years.[6]

Theologians are not sure what the scripture meant here when it says
that, "the sons of God saw that the daughters of men were beautiful".
Some think that it meant that a race of angels bred with the women of
mankind. Some think that the people of faith bred with those without
faith. One thing is clear from this passage. God decided that because
of the choices man was making, He must limit the age of mankind so
that the violence and disobedience would not totally destroy mankind.
The violence became so bad that God was sorry that He had made
mankind and decided to end it all, except for one man and his family.

> And GOD saw that the wickedness of man *was* great in the
> earth, and *that* every imagination of the thoughts of his heart
> *was* only evil continually. And it repented the LORD that he
> had made man on the earth, and it grieved him at his heart.
> And the LORD said, I will destroy man whom I have created
> from the face of the earth; both man, and beast, and the
> creeping thing, and the fowls of the air; for it repenteth me
> that I have made them. But Noah found grace in the eyes of
> the LORD. [7]

AN END TO DIVINE PATIENCE

Some may question whether this world was ever really perfect because of the growth of violence from its beginnings. But we must remember that it was not God who committed the first sin, it was man, who had been given a free will. Free will is a love gift. It is a gift that makes us truly independent. Mankind has not been programmed into blind obedience. We have choices that are totally up to us. Of course God knows what choices we will make before we are ever faced with them. The agape love of the Lord Jesus Christ flowers in our gift of free choice. Yet, free choice leads us into error because we are sinful and rebellious ever since that day in the perfect garden.

The free will of mankind has always been a problem for our Creator. He loves us and wants us to love Him of our own free will, but we are bound and determined to do our own selfish will. Why God allows sin is a great mystery. I believe that He has allowed us to sin, because that is the only way for us to love Him freely. Sin leads us into all kinds of trouble and eventually into death. That is why God's perfect plan had to include the sacrifice of His only Son to pay our sin debt. When we realize that God loved us so much that He gave us freedom to love or reject Him; when we realize that He loves us even though we deserve death and hell; when we realize that only through the precious blood of His only Son can we have eternal forgiveness; then I believe that we should bow to our knees and even prostrate ourselves on our faces and confess that we are sinners and need forgiveness from a Holy God. Repentance from sin and a surrender to God's perfect will come from a contrite and broken heart, a heart that loves God for who He is and for what He has done for us.

So God decided that because mankind was awesome and powerful, large and cunning, but hopelessly sinful and violent, He must start over and wipe the slate clean. God found that one man had kept himself clean and been obedient through all the temptation that had come. That man was Noah. Surely Noah was not sinless, but the Lord saw in him the rekindling of a spirit of love for the Father. God knew that there was only one hope for mankind and that hope was Noah and his family.

PRELUDE TO DELUGE

As men grew in numbers and strength in the post-Eden world, God became more and more regretful that He had made man.

God didn't make a mistake when he made mankind or the animals or the rest of creation. The mistake was man's, not God's. It was God who was disappointed that man couldn't or wouldn't discipline himself to love and obedience. It was God who was saddened that His creation chose to disregard the love and provision that had been carefully lavished upon it. Just as it grieves an earthly father to see his children make mistakes of judgment and character, I believe that God in a similar manner saw that His children were making mistake after mistake leading to deeper and deeper depravity, and so He decided to shorten their lifespan.

But there was one man in whom God saw possibilities. That man was Noah. Noah found grace in the eyes of the Lord and was spared along with his family. God told Noah how to build the Ark and for years Noah and his sons worked on it. Can you imagine the things that the people said to Noah for building such a huge vessel and preaching that it was going to rain water from the sky, when it had never rained? But, sure enough, God sent the rain and told Noah and his family to get into the Ark.

> And Noah *was* six hundred years old when the flood of waters was upon the earth. And Noah went in, and his sons, and his wife, and his sons' wives with him, into the ark, because of the waters of the flood. Of clean beasts, and of beasts that *are* not clean, and of fowls, and of every thing that creepeth upon the earth, There went in two and two unto Noah into the ark, the male and the female, as God had commanded Noah. And it came to pass after seven days, that the waters of the flood were upon the earth.

> In the six hundredth year of Noah's life, in the second month, the seventeenth day of the month, the same day were all the fountains of the great deep broken up, and the windows of heaven were opened. And the rain was upon the earth forty days and forty nights.[8]

The moment they were in the Ark the canopy broke, the fountains of the deep opened up and water, snow, and ice began covering the entire earth. The giants of the earth didn't have a chance. They were drowned, frozen, and buried in seas of mud and silt. Imagine the heaviest rain you've ever seen, and then imagine that the ground started belching out water that had been locked below for hundreds of years. In only forty days, the whole earth was submerged and the only living things that breathed were the animals and Noah's family on the Ark. All trees, plants, and air-breathing animals were quickly killed and deposited in layers over all the earth, leaving deposits of carbon that thousands of years later would be sucked out of the ground as crude oil and gas. Carcasses of both the titan and the tiny were woven into the sediment of the giant sea.

One model suggested by a creation scientist is that God could have sent a comet to hit the earth causing the flood. This could account for the canopy being damaged and the earth's axis to be tilted 23 1/2 degrees, thus causing seasons of summer, fall, winter, and spring. This would also explain the ice age, where the polar caps expanded drastically over a short period of time and gradually receded. Another model suggests that the polar ice caps could have proceeded and receded in just a few years rather than in a few hundred thousand.

After one year on the worldwide sea, the big boat touched land on Mount Ararat, and the only remaining humans walked out of the Ark. All vegetation had been drowned or frozen so there was nothing to eat. But what did Noah do? Did he get hungry and start slaughtering the animals for food? No! He built an altar and sacrificed from every clean beast and every clean fowl that was on the Ark. This is the first recorded burnt offering. The Lord saw that Noah had sacrificed the very best animals on the ark as a love offering of thankfulness, and faithfulness, trusting that God would provide for them. I believe that Noah realized that instead of shedding his blood, God had spared him and his family. God was pleased with the sacrifice and made new rules for the new world.

> And the LORD smelled a sweet savour; and the LORD said
> in his heart, I will not again curse the ground any more for
> man's sake; for the imagination of man's heart *is* evil from

his youth; neither will I again smite any more every thing living, as I have done. While the earth remaineth, seedtime and harvest, and cold and heat, and summer and winter, and day and night shall not cease.[9]

---

[1]*The Holy Bible : King James Version.*, Ps 32:1. Oak Harbor, WA: Logos Research Systems, Inc., 1995.

[2]*The Holy Bible : King James Version.*, 1 Co 15:21. Oak Harbor, WA: Logos Research Systems, Inc., 1995.

[3]*The Holy Bible : King James Version.*, Ge 3:22-24. Oak Harbor, WA: Logos Research Systems, Inc., 1995.

[4] *New Naves Topical Bible: 1994 Revised*, Logos Research Systems Incorporated, James Swanson.

[5]*The Holy Bible : King James Version.*, Ge 5:23-24. Oak Harbor, WA: Logos Research Systems, Inc., 1995.

[6]*The Holy Bible : King James Version.*, Ge 6:1-3. Oak Harbor, WA: Logos Research Systems, Inc., 1995.

[7]*The Holy Bible : King James Version.*, Ge 6:5-8. Oak Harbor, WA: Logos Research Systems, Inc., 1995.

[8]*The Holy Bible : King James Version.*, Ge 7:6-12. Oak Harbor, WA: Logos Research Systems, Inc., 1995.

[9]*The Holy Bible : King James Version.*, Ge 8:20-22. Oak Harbor, WA: Logos Research Systems, Inc., 1995.

CHAPTER 3

P L A N   B

THE NEW WORLD

This new world that now had a total of eight humans and a small number of animals and plants began the impossible task of replenishing the earth. God told them to "Be fruitful and multiply, and replenish the earth". Somehow that command has been watered down in this day of "the pill" and "family planning". But how could this new world survive without any vegetation to feed the living animals? God provided the answer in the next chapter.

> And God blessed Noah and his sons, and said unto them, Be fruitful, and multiply, and replenish the earth. And the fear of you and the dread of you shall be upon every beast of the earth, and upon every fowl of the air, upon all that moveth *upon* the earth, and upon all the fishes of the sea; into your hand are they delivered. Every moving thing that liveth shall be meat for you; even as the green herb have I given you all things.[1]

For the second time God commanded mankind to be fruitful and multiply. But how could they survive in this new beginning? Everything had changed! The water canopy had been almost completely destroyed. The green earth was replaced by vast oceans. The sea of air that living things dwelled in had less pressure and less oxygen, resulting in faster aging and more harmful radiation from the sun. The earth wobbled on its axis and polar ice caps quickly formed and then melted away, carving the earth in the process. This twenty-three and one-half degree wobble caused seasons of alternating cold and hot. Some areas of the world were now very hostile to plant growth year-round. Rainfall was necessary for sustained growth and maturation.

Up until now the animals had no fear of man because man did not hunt the animals for food because there were plenty of green plants to eat. But because of the need for food for mankind, God relaxed His perfect diet to accommodate the survival of His chosen vessel. God's perfect will was set aside and His permissive will was instituted. In one verse the whole order of life on earth was changed and man became the hunter. Have you ever noticed that animals have an inborn fear of mankind? The domesticated animals have overcome that fear to some extent, but wild animals have an instinctive fear and dread of man because of God's change in the fabric of creation.

However, there was one stipulation to the eating of animals. They were not to abuse the right to kill and eat. There would be respect for life even in killing for food and the lifeblood of the animals was not to be consumed.

> But flesh with the life thereof, *which is* the blood thereof, shall ye not eat. And surely your blood of your lives will I require; at the hand of every beast will I require it, and at the hand of man; at the hand of every man's brother will I require the life of man. Whoso sheddeth man's blood, by man shall his blood be shed: for in the image of God made he man.[2]

God changed His rules to accommodate an imperfect creation. His perfect will gives way to His permissive will. Killing would be under strict guidelines. Even wild animals kill their prey and bleed it before eating it. This passage also gives authority to mankind to take the life of one who kills another without justification.

You must keep in mind that this new start or new genesis was instituted as punishment for the sin of mankind. Thus, there are curses that we must live under that were not present in the Garden. First and foremost is the curse of death. God instituted death because it is the punishment for sin against a perfectly holy God. This curse is realized because the new environment promotes death and results in death. God does not allow us to have eternal physical life here on this earth in its present form. How did God limit the lifespan of mankind? In several ways:

THREE DRASTIC CHANGES

First, God has **limited our lifespan** by narrowing the gene pool to eight humans, thus allowing the loss of the long-life mechanism that enables humans to live hundreds of years. The gene pool of the eight remaining humans was severely limited and we lost the long-life genes that Noah and his ancestors had enjoyed. Other factors that limit our lifespan are weather, atmospheric gases, radiation, and diet.

Secondly, God has **limited our liveliness** by giving us meat and by changing our environment. There is a positive side of this new law and a negative side. On the positive side, we are allowed to kill animals and eat their flesh for survival and enjoyment. On the negative side, we are destined for early death by eating the flesh of animals because it is a death-promoting diet. Animal flesh, including animal milk and animal eggs, were not the intended diet for humans or animals. It is not a sin to eat animal products. But it is an act that limits our liveliness and our lifespan, just as intended by God.

After following the most rigorous scientific rules of research, Dr. T. Colin Campbell found that "dietary protein proved to be so powerful in its effect that we could turn on and turn off cancer growth simply by changing the level consumed."

> But that's not all. We found that not all proteins had this effect. What protein consistently and strongly promoted cancer? Casein, which makes up 87% of cow's milk protein, promoted all stages of the cancer process. What type of protein did not promote cancer, even at high levels of intake? The safe proteins were from plants, including wheat and soy. As this picture came into view, it began to challenge and then to shatter some of my most cherished assumptions (that meat and dairy products were healthy).[3]

We are also no longer in a perfect environment, as in the Garden where there were no harmful microbes, deadly radiation, extreme weather, polluted air and water, man-eating animals, and sin in the heart of mankind. These two changes cause us to lose good health long before the 120-year limit to our physical lives.

Thirdly, God has **limited our living with Him**. He no longer walks with us and talks with us person to person as He did with Adam. He speaks now indirectly through His inspired word and by His Holy Spirit. This is a blessing, but also a curse in that we don't have direct personal contact with our Creator. This limits our lifespan by opening up to us to all kinds of deadly choices. Because He is not constantly at our side, we are repeatedly tripping over life-threatening choices on the road of life.

> Therefore we are always confident, knowing that, whilst we are at home in the body, we are absent from the Lord: 7 (For we walk by faith, not by sight:) 8 We are confident, I say, and willing rather to be absent from the body, and to be present with the Lord.[4]

What were the results of this change? Noah and his family started eating meat and the lifespan of mankind dropped from the 900's to the 90's in a matter of decades. No longer would the water canopy protect man. No longer would he breathe high-pressure oxygen and live in stable weather conditions. Now the earth wobbled on its axis and seasons began to wax and wane as did the tides of the sea. Creature hunted creature. Fear gripped the earth. This was the new world – cold and cruel.

REIGNING IN THE REBELLIOUS

Did man get better for having been spared annihilation? Did he learn his lesson? Was this a better world after the washing with water? Over three hundred years after the flood ended, God saw that mankind had not changed and that again He must intervene to keep mankind from self- destruction.

And the whole earth was of one language, and of one speech. And it came to pass, as they journeyed from the east, that they found a plain in the land of Shinar; and they dwelt there. And they said one to another, Go to, let us make brick, and burn them thoroughly. And they had brick for stone, and slime had they for morter. And they said, Go to, let us build us a city and a tower, whose top *may reach* unto heaven; and let us make us a name, lest we be scattered abroad upon the face of the whole earth. And the LORD came down to see the city and the tower, which the children of men builded. And the LORD said, Behold, the people *is* one, and they have all one language; and this they begin to do: and now nothing will be restrained from them, which they have imagined to do. Go to, let us go down, and there confound their language, that they may not understand one another's speech. So the LORD scattered them abroad from thence upon the face of all the earth: and they left off to build the city. Therefore is the name of it called Babel; because the LORD did there confound the language of all the earth: and from thence did the LORD scatter them abroad upon the face of all the earth.[5]

God is perfect and holy. He does not change. He has been, is, and will always be perfect and holy. But because He is love, He also allows free will. His holiness caused Him to destroy much of the sinful world that had multiplied. His love allowed mankind to continue in a less than perfect world. For survival in this new world, they would have to kill animals for food. Disease would be a natural result of this new lifestyle. Finally, God's perfect plan of a righteous nation over all the earth was spoiled by man's pride. The result was God's righteous judgment to confuse and scatter rather than to allow further decadence.

PLAN B

The Battle Plan B for dietary health is for man to eat meat if he can't eat the plant foods he needs. **But Plan B is not the optimum for health. It is for survival and for sacrificial symbolism, and our sentence for sin.** Christians have taken God's permission to eat meat to the extreme. We live in a world where killing animals has reached a cold, calculated

art.   Americans have killed senselessly and eaten glutinously and
suffered the consequences.

Now more than ever, America is a nation of meat eaters. In
2000, total meat consumption (red meat, poultry, and fish)
reached 195 pounds (boneless, trimmed-weight equivalent)
per person , 57 pounds above-average annual consumption in
the 1950s. Each American consumed an average of 7 pounds
more red meat than in the 1950s, 46 pounds more poultry,
and 4 pounds more fish and shellfish.[6]

**Our lust for flesh has brought us down to lower depths than
ever before. God lovingly allowed us to eat meat for survival, but
we have perverted this freedom into a massacre of gigantic
proportions.** Americans eat meat at every meal and are insensitive to
the suffering of animals that have provided that hamburger, hot dog,
pizza, steak, and chicken sandwich.   Pulitzer Prize nominee, John
Robbins, in his book The Food Revolution, states that "More animals
are being subjected to more torturous conditions in the United States
today than has ever occurred anywhere in world history."

B FOR BRUTALITY

Most people think that animals are dead before they are cut into pieces,
but this is not always the case. In his book, The Food Revolution, John
Robbins relates that instances where cows are hoisted by their hind
legs, skinned and slaughtered while they are still alive have been
documented on video. Affidavits from slaughter house employees have
testified to the fact that thousands of cows went through the slaughter
process alive and that their supervisors required them to work on cows
that were still alive.[7] Chickens are jammed into wire cages with no
exercise or sunshine, fed growth hormones, and brought to slaughter by
the end of eight weeks of age. Baby calves are kept in tight quarters and
slaughtered at a few months of age for popular veal. Brutality of this
sort is more common than we would like to believe. And the state of
affairs in America is much worse than in the rest of the world.

"Attorney David Wolfson commented, 'The contrast is stark: the United States alters the law to allow cruel farming practices while Western European countries are banning cruel farming practices."[8]

I believe that most Americans, including livestock farmers, have little knowledge of this state of affairs in the slaughter industry. When we order our hamburger, pizza, chicken fingers, or baby back ribs, we have little thought of what suffering the animal endured to satisfy our appetite for pleasure. The demand for the lives of 90,000 cows every 24 hours, 14,000 chickens per minute, and 10 billion food animals per year in the United States testifies to our gluttony and degradation. Could we survive without this gargantuan slaughter? The question should be "Why do we continue this unnecessary brutality when we have a much healthier and life-promoting option of fruits and vegetables, nuts and seeds?"

BETTER BUT NOT BEST

It doesn't take a PhD to figure out that the people groups that eat a plant-based diet are much healthier than people groups that eat animal products. Just visit such places as rural China, India, or any other developing nation or people group that eats a plant-based diet. You'll find that the degenerative diseases that are rampant in the U.S., Britain, Sweden, and other highly developed countries are virtually non-existent in the countries that eat a primarily plant-based diet.

The animals, including their entire bodies, were given to us for our benefit. They have no spirit and are not made in God's image. But is it right to brutalize them and make them suffer just to satisfy our selfish appetites? In this twenty first century mankind has again perverted a freedom into a license. A plant-based diet is easily achievable even in this cursed world. But our insatiable appetite for flesh has led us into a cruel and unholy massacre of millions of animals. It is no wonder that violation of God's natural dietary law has unleashed upon us deadly diseases that are largely a result of our insatiable appetite for flesh. The diseases that kill us began after the flood and continue today. The Bible contains hundreds of instances of diseases brought on by the desire for flesh.

DISEASES AFTER THE DELUGE

The post-diluvian age brought with it toxicity and diseases, such as barrenness (Gen. 18:12), boils (II Kings 20:7), blindness (Matt. 8:22, John 9:1), consumption (Deut. 28:22), deafness (Lev. 19:14), dropsy (Luke 14:2), dumbness (Matt. 7:32), dysentery (II Chronicles 21:18), epilepsy (Matt. 4:24), fever (Deut. 28:22, Luke 4:38), gout (II Chronicles 16:12), hemophilia (Matt. 9:18), leprosy (Lev. 13:18, Luke 17:12), mental disorder (Ecclesiastes 9:3), menorrhagia (Mark 5:25), palsy (Luke 5:17), plague (Exodus 9:3), poliomyelitis, (Matthew 12:10), prolapsed rectum (2 Chronicles 21:15, 18-19), scabs (Leviticus 21:20), sterility (Genesis 16:1, Genesis 30:1, Luke 1:25), tumors (1 Samuel 5:6), and wen or warts (Leviticus 22:22).[9]

LIES THAT HAVE LULLED US

Yet with these effects tied directly to animal products, we still deny the cause.   The food and drug industry's pressure on government bureaucracy, coupled with the consent of traditional medicine, has led us to believe lies such as:

"Milk (pasteurized cow milk) is necessary for strong bones and teeth."

The Harvard Nurses' Health Study of 77,761 women, aged 34 to 59 followed for 12 years, found that those who drank three or more glasses of milk per day had no reduction in the risk of hip or arm fractures compared to those who drank little or no milk, even after adjustment for weight, menopausal status, smoking, and alcohol use. In fact, the fracture rates were slightly, but significantly, higher for those who consumed this much milk, compared to those who drank little or no milk.[10]

"Meat is the only source of essential amino acids for health. Plants do not have all the nutrients necessary for human health."

"Any combination of natural foods will supply you with adequate protein, including all eight essential amino acids as well as unessential amino acids." Dr. Joel Fuhrman[11]

"I now consider veganism to be the ideal diet. A vegan (no animal products) diet — particularly one that is low in fat — will substantially reduce disease risks. Plus, we've seen no disadvantages from veganism." Dr. T. Colin Campbell[12]

The new U.S.D.A. web site for updated Food Pyramid and Food Guidelines acknowledges that:

"Vegetarian diets can meet all the recommendations for nutrients."[13]

"Our government makes sure that animal products are safe for consumption."

"Currrently, we have over 100 million head of cattle in the US and in the last thirteen years we have only tested 57,000 animals for mad cow disease. France has 11 million cattle in their herd and they test 66,000 each week. I believe in the US we have had a "don't look, don't find" policy and up until the 23rd of December, it worked." Howard Lyman, author of <u>Mad Cowboy</u>, speaking from his web site in January 2004.[14]

The Center for Disease Control (CDC) calculates that every year in the United States, there are approximately 76 million cases of food-borne illness, with 325,000 hospitalizations and 5,000 deaths. These statistics represent all cases of food-borne illness, not simply those spread by meat and poultry. The CDC does not provide statistics breaking down cases of food-borne illness by their source, but as reported in "Modern Meat," it is estimated that at least one third of the 5,000 deaths each year from food-borne illness can be attributed to meat and poultry.[15]

"Osteoporosis, Diabetes, Heart Disease, Cancer, and Arthritis are incurable diseases."

Plant-based nutrition provides us with a pathway to escape the coronary artery disease epidemic. For persons in central Africa, the Papua Highlanders of New Guinea, the Tarahumara Indians of northern Mexico, and inhabitants of rural China as described in the Cornell China Study, coronary disease is essentially non-existent while hypertension, Western malignancies, obesity, and adult-onset diabetes are rarely encountered.[16]

"The War on Cancer will be won by spending more money on research to find a cure."

NCCR, a coalition of 26 national research and lay advocacy organizations working to secure adequate federal funding for research to improve cancer prevention, detection, treatment, and survivorship, is concerned that 42% of Americans will develop cancer and 25% will die of cancer, with costs exceeding $107 billion this year alone. Conservative estimates project that by 2010 cancer will become the leading cause of death as incidence increases 29% and mortality 25% at an annual cost of over $200 billion.[17]

"The World Health Organization has carried out the first ever analysis of the world's health systems. The findings are published 21 June, 2000, in The World Health Report 2000 – Health systems: Improving performance.
The U. S. health system spends a higher portion of its gross domestic product than any other country but ranks 37 out of 191 countries according to its performance, the report finds."[18]

---

1 *The Holy Bible : King James Version.*, Ge 9:1-3. Oak Harbor, WA: Logos Research Systems, Inc., 1995.
2 *The Holy Bible : King James Version.*, Ge 9:4-6. Oak Harbor, WA: Logos Research Systems, Inc., 1995.
3 Campbell, T. Colin, *The China Study* (Dallas: Benbella Books, 2005), 6.
4 2 Corinthians 5:6-8. KJV

[5] *The Holy Bible : King James Version.*, Ge 11:1-9. Oak Harbor, WA: Logos Research Systems, Inc., 1995.

[6] http://www.usda.gov/factbook/chapter2.htm

[7] Robbins, John. *The Food Revolution* Conari Press. Berkeley CA. 2001, p.211.

[8] Robbins, John. The Food Revolution. Canari Press. Berkeley CA. 2001

[9] The New Bible Dictionary. Third Edition. Intervarsity Press. England. P. 446.

[10] http://www.pcrm.org/resources/education/nutrition/nutrition7.htmlFeskanich D, Willett WC, Stampfer MJ, Colditz GA. Milk, dietary calcium, and bone fractures in women: a 12-year prospective study. Am J Publ Health 1997;87:992-7.

[11] Furhman, Joel. Eat to Live. Little, Brown, and Co. Boston, New York, London. 2003.

[12] http://www.gentleworld.org/health/health.html. Campbell, T. Colin. The China Project.

[13] http://www.mypyramid.gov/tips_resources/vegetarian_diets_print.html

[14] Lyman, Howard. http://www.madcowboy.com/02_HowardMCusa.html

[15] http://www.pbs.org/wgbh/pages/frontline/shows/meat/safe/foodborne.html.

[16] Esselstyne, Caldwell, Jr., M.D. *September 2, 2000 in Orlando, Florida at the Summit Conference on Cholesterol and Coronary Risk presented by the Cleveland Clinic Foundation in cooperation with the Walt Disney World Company.*

[17] http://www.cancercoalition.org/priorities.html. The National Coalition for Cancer Research, Legislative Update, Washington, D.C., July, 2004.

[18] http://www.photius.com/rankings/who_world_health_ranks.html

CHAPTER 4

SACRIFICE VS. OBEDIENCE

To Obey is Better Than Sacrifice

One of the most misunderstood concepts in the Bible is the difference between sacrifices and obedience. There was no need for sacrifices in the Garden because there was no sin. There was nothing to make up for or to owe. No sin, no consequences. Sin, on the other hand, has a very high price and must be recompensed. Sin against a holy and just God has consequences that are automatic and eternal. King Saul disobeyed God when told by the Lord through the prophet, Samuel, to totally wipe out the Amalekites. Saul spared the king and some of the animals to offer a sacrifice to the Lord.

> And Samuel said, Hath the LORD as great delight in burnt offerings and sacrifices, as in obeying the voice of the LORD? Behold, to obey is better than sacrifice, and to hearken than the fat of rams.[1]

The very first sin by Adam and Eve resulted in eternal separation from God. Today, our sin separates us from God. Only through the precious blood of the Lamb of God, Jesus Christ, is there payment for sin and restored fellowship and acceptance by our Creator and Savior. And one must accept that sacrifice and surrender to Him as Lord and Saviour in order to be cleansed, once and for all, of sins past, present, and future.

And almost all things are by the law purged with blood; and
without shedding of blood is no remission.[2]

SACRIFICIAL SYMBOLISM

There is and has always been only one payment for sin and that has
always been life blood. God instituted sacrifices to show mankind that
sin has a very high price. Animals are precious in God's sight. They
are His workmanship and are very close to being in His image, although
they lack a spirit. The first sacrifice was instituted by God for Adam and
Eve so that they might have clothing.

> Unto Adam also and to his wife did the LORD God make
> coats of skins, and clothed them.[3]

Just as an earthly father is honored by his children's obedience and
reverence, so our heavenly Father is honored by his children's
obedience and reverence. There is no need for making up for
disobedience when there is obedience. A sacrifice is not necessary if no
sin has required it.

To teach man about sin and sacrificial blood atonement, God instituted
animal sacrifices in the Garden of Eden when He demonstrated that sin
results in death, in this case the death of an animal to cover their
nakedness (Genesis 3:21). The deeper meaning was that the sin sacrifice
was to represent the final sacrifice of God's Son Jesus as the only
atonement for sin.

> What can wash away my sin?
> Nothing but the blood of Jesus;
> What can make me whole again?
> Nothing but the blood of Jesus.
>
> Oh! precious is the flow
> That makes me white as snow;
> No other fount I know,
> Nothing but the blood of Jesus.[4]

God killed the first animal as a sacrifice for man's sin. The faithful followed this practice right up until the final sacrifice, the Lord Jesus Christ. Until that precious blood was spilt, no sacrifice was enough to pay for sin. God used the blood of animals to show that sin has a price that can only be paid by the taking of a life. In the case of Cain and Abel's offerings, God demonstrated that the perfect offering would be a sacrifice of first-born and not first fruits (Gen. 4:3-5).

EAT TO LIVE

Noah offered the first burnt offering, in which the entire animal was sacrificed as an acknowledgement of God as Provider and Saviour, even in the face of starvation. The world was a very unfriendly place just after the flood subsided, and as a result of the devastation of all plant life, there was little if any plant life to eat. I believe that God allowed mankind to eat animal flesh to remind us that without the shedding of blood there is no life. The Lord Jesus also told His disciples that life only came from eating His flesh and drinking His blood.

> Verily, verily, I say unto you, Except ye eat the flesh of the Son of man, and drink his blood, ye have no life in you. Whoso eateth my flesh, and drinketh my blood, hath eternal life; and I will raise him up at the last day. For my flesh is meat indeed, and my blood is drink indeed. He that eateth my flesh, and drinketh my blood, dwelleth in me, and I in him. As the living Father hath sent me, and I live by the Father: so he that eateth me, even he shall live by me. This is that bread which came down from heaven: not as your fathers did eat manna, and are dead: he that eateth of this bread shall live for ever. These things said he in the synagogue, as he taught in Capernaum.[5]

Aaron, Moses' brother, became the first priest in his line, and they all practiced sacrificial offerings to make up for the trespasses against a Holy God. As part of these rituals, recorded in Leviticus, the priests were allowed to eat portions of the sacrificial animals. God was careful to demand that the fat, the tastiest but also the most deadly part of an animal, was to be burned up entirely as a sweet smell to the Lord. This practice continued up until the coming of Messiah, Jesus, the Christ, the final sacrifice. The last supper was preceded by the Pascal meal when the Passover lamb was sacrificed, roasted, and eaten.

DEVOTED DISCIPLINE

But what about the alternative? Is there a way to avoid having to sacrifice a life? Yes, there is! And that alternative is obedience. **Just as Adam and Eve were obedient to the God of Creation, we can be obedient also and avoid the taking of a life. That life is our own!** No, we cannot avoid the sin that is a part of our being. All Christians have sinned, are sinning, and will continue to sin because we have a sin nature. But we can die to sin daily and take up our cross and follow Jesus. Christians can be obedient in taking care of their bodies and can avoid or postpone the end result of death and disease. Maybe we can't live to be 900, but we can live to be 120 and more. There are remote peoples who live to be over 100 years old and more on plant foods.

How can Christians live longer and healthier? How do we avoid sickness, disease, lack of energy, dementia, and other signs of physical degeneration? By being obedient in our eating habits, drinking habits, and lifestyle habits, we can extend our life-spans and increase our effectiveness in living for Christ Jesus.

RETURN TO RESPONSIBILITY

The alternative to gluttony and disease is obedience to the original plant-based diet of Eden. Time and time again the plant-based diet has shown to be the lifestyle of health and wellness, as well as the diet of longevity. According to the AARP, the average lifespan of Americans is only 77.2 years, and many of those are sick and weak long before their death. For many thousands of Americans who are on plant-based diets, there is escape from the consequences of undisciplined eating and drinking. The elimination of animal flesh and their by-products from our diet can result in much better health and wellness for as long as we live. This voluntary sanctification of our body temples through a plant-based diet can lead to vitality and wellness not attainable through a meat-based diet.

The life of an animal and mankind is in the blood. The life of a plant is in its juice, containing chlorophyll. The chlorophyll molecule in plants is very similar to the hemoglobin molecule in blood. The only difference is that instead of having iron in it the chlorophyll molecule has a magnesium atom in it. The juice of plants contains the nutrition that the body must have for life. That is why juicing is such a beneficial part of a healthy diet. Instead of the body expending energy to separate the juice from the fiber, machines do the job. Then the juice, with concentrated nutrition can go to cell level and multiply the effect of life giving plant fluids on the body.

FROM SLAVERY TO SANCTIFICATION

Some of the most illuminating scripture references dealing with diet are the experiences of the Israelites during their exodus from Egyptian slavery. In Egypt the Israelites were well fed. The rich Nile Valley had provided a wide variety of fruits and vegetables, nuts and seeds, fish, beef, lamb and other delicacies that even slaves were occasionally able to enjoy. As told in Exodus 16, Israel had marched into the desert only one month's journey when the people started complaining about the lack of water, meat, and vegetables they had enjoyed back in Egypt. Makes you wonder what happened to all the livestock they had with them. Were they so disciplined that they wouldn't eat the livestock because they were saving it for sacrifices? Could be. It could be that they were saving their livestock for the Promised Land and it was their life savings for a better future. Another plausible explanation is that the Israelites knew that a diet of only meat was an unhealthy diet that would result in disease and ill health. In Egypt they had enjoyed lots of fresh vegetables, fruits, nuts and seeds. In the wilderness there were no such luxuries. Almost immediately the people grumbled.

> And they took their journey from Elim, and all the congregation of the children of Israel came unto the wilderness of Sin, which *is* between Elim and Sinai, on the fifteenth day of the second month after their departing out of the land of Egypt. And the whole congregation of the children of Israel murmured against Moses and Aaron in the wilderness: And the children of Israel said unto them, Would to God we had died by the hand of the LORD in the land of

Egypt, when we sat by the flesh pots, *and* when we did eat bread to the full; for ye have brought us forth into this wilderness, to kill this whole assembly with hunger. Then said the LORD unto Moses, Behold, I will rain bread from heaven for you; and the people shall go out and gather a certain rate every day, that I may prove them, whether they will walk in my law, or no. And it shall come to pass, that on the sixth day they shall prepare *that* which they bring in; and it shall be twice as much as they gather daily.[6]

MIRACLE MANNA

In the wilderness of Sin at the eighth encampment the Israelites were given manna from God. It looked like coriander seed, tasted like cakes made with honey, and lasted only one day, except when gathered on the day before the Sabbath it lasted two days. It could be baked or boiled, ground in mills, or beaten in a mortar. It was truly a miracle food straight from God. Matthew Henry explains manna from Numbers 11 this way.

It was bread from heaven, angels' food. To show how unreasonable their complaint was, it is here described, v. 7-9. It was good for food, and pleasant to the eye, every grain like an orient pearl; it was wholesome food and nourishing; it was not to be called *dry bread,* for it tasted like fresh oil; it was agreeable (the Jews say, Wisd. 16:20) to every man's palate, and tasted as he would have it; and, though it was still the same, yet, by the different ways of dressing it, it yielded them a grateful variety; it cost them no money, nor care, for it fell in the night, while they slept; and the labour of gathering it was not worth speaking of; they lived upon free quarter, and yet could talk of Egypt's cheapness and the fish they ate there freely. Nay, which was much more valuable than all this, the manna came from the immediate power and bounty of God, not from common providence, but from special favour. It was, as God's compassion, new every morning, always fresh, not as their food who live on shipboard. While they lived on manna, they seemed to be exempted from the curse which sin has brought on man, that in the *sweat of his face should he eat bread.* And yet they speak of manna with such scorn, as if it were not good enough to be meat for swine: *Our soul is dried away.* They speak as if God dealt hardly with them in allowing them no better food.[7]

LIVESTOCK FUTURES

The Israelites did not slaughter their livestock, which was their future, for food. They would use the livestock only for sacrifices later to be instituted in the Tabernacle worship. We don't know how the livestock were fed but it must have been another miracle from the Lord to feed all those sheep, cattle, and oxen with manna. The Israelites ate manna for the entire forty years in the wilderness until they entered the Promised Land. God only gave them meat on two occasions, here in Exodus and then again in Numbers 11.

> And it came to pass, that at even the quails came up, and covered the camp: and in the morning the dew lay round about the host. And when the dew that lay was gone up, behold, upon the face of the wilderness *there lay* a small round thing, *as* small as the hoar frost on the ground. And when the children of Israel saw *it*, they said one to another, It *is* manna: for they wist not what it *was*. And Moses said unto them, This *is* the bread which the LORD hath given you to eat.[8]

In Exodus 17 we find that the people also murmured against God because of the lack of water. God gave them water in a miraculous way, using again the rod that had divided the waters of the Red Sea.

> And the LORD said unto Moses, Go on before the people, and take with thee of the elders of Israel; and thy rod, wherewith thou smotest the river, take in thine hand, and go. Behold, I will stand before thee there upon the rock in Horeb; and thou shalt smite the rock, and there shall come water out of it, that the people may drink.[9]

The miracles of the exodus began when God provided food and water for them in the desert. God had given the Israelites approximately 240 boxcar loads of manna a day (Exodus 16). This food was perfect and balanced nutrition created by the Creator for His people. Over 2 million Jews took up over 7.2 square miles of desert for just themselves, not counting their livestock. It took several hundred average backyard swimming pools of water to allow one gallon of water per Israelite per day. So the miracles of the Exodus were numerous to say the least. [10]

CARROTS FOR COMPLIANCE

God promised the Israelites much reward for obedience. His blessings are spiritual and physical, intangible and tangible, evident and hidden. Like a father who favors an obedient and respectful son over a rebellious and impertinent one, God rewards reverence and discipline and love.

> If ye walk in my statutes, and keep my commandments, and do them; Then I will give you rain in due season, and the land shall yield her increase, and the trees of the field shall yield their fruit. And your threshing shall reach unto the vintage, and the vintage shall reach unto the sowing time: and ye shall eat your bread to the full, and dwell in your land safely. And I will give peace in the land, and ye shall lie down, and none shall make *you* afraid: and I will rid evil beasts out of the land, neither shall the sword go through your land. And ye shall chase your enemies, and they shall fall before you by the sword. And five of you shall chase an hundred, and an hundred of you shall put ten thousand to flight: and your enemies shall fall before you by the sword. For I will have respect unto you, and make you fruitful, and multiply you, and establish my covenant with you. And ye shall eat old store, and bring forth the old because of the new. And I will set my tabernacle among you: and my soul shall not abhor you. And I will walk among you, and will be your God, and ye shall be my people. I *am* the LORD your God, which brought you forth out of the land of Egypt, that ye should not be their bondmen; and I have broken the bands of your yoke, and made you go upright. [11]

Here we see into the mind and heart of God toward His children, toward those whom He has called as heirs to His kingdom. Here we see that in God's perfect plan for obedient children there is no need for killing, no need for shedding of blood of animals or of man. He promised them rain just when it was needed for crops. He promised trees full of fruit. He promised that there would be no span between crops or harvests. The old crop would be plentiful until the new crop could be harvested. God would feed his obedient children all they could eat and they would be strong and protected by His mighty hand. His promise toward obedient children was that they would not be afraid of anything including wild beasts, harmful insects, nor violent people. We are promised plentiful crops of food consisting of grain, fruits, vegetables – BUT NOT MEAT. Why did God give the Israelites quail on only two occasions and manna for the entire forty years in the wilderness? Because manna was perfect food and the meat of animals was detrimental to their health. The permissive will of God allows animal flesh for survival while the perfect will of God yields blessings of healthy plant nutrition upon which our miraculous bodies flourish.

SANCTIFIED SACRIFICES

After God gave Moses the law on Mt. Sinai, He also gave him the law of the sacrifices and the law of unclean and clean animals. Actually, the concept of clean and unclean animals was first given in Genesis 7:2 where God specified that Noah take seven clean pairs of animals into the ark and only one pair of unclean animals. Then in Mosaic law of Leviticus 11-15 and again in Numbers 19 we find instructions against eating of unclean flesh. In the case of swine, the Israelites did not know that trichinosis was a very deadly parasite transmitted by inadequate cooking of the meat. It is probable that other unknown dangers lurked in the meat of these other animals that God commanded that His people avoid. Aquatic animals that did not have fins or scales were expressly forbidden since they were scavengers. Even birds of prey were not allowed as sacrifices or to be eaten.

Even of the clean animals there were restrictions as to which parts of the clean animals were unclean. The fat of the intestines, the fat of the kidneys, and the fat of the tail were expressly prohibited in Exodus 29:13 and 22, in Leviticus 3:4-9; 9:19; 17:10; and 19:26. God expressly

forbade His people from eating the dangerous animal fats that would
lead to sickness and early death. Although animal fat is very delicious,
as evidenced by marbled beef in prime rib, it is also very detrimental to
health.

UNGRATEFUL GRUMBLERS

In Numbers 11 God again is blamed for the troubles of His disobedient
children. Having been provided with manna, water, light, and heat, and
having been spared from hostile people and swelling feet and tattered
clothing, some of God's children again became murmurers and
complainers. They craved meat once again. And this time even Moses
grumbled that he had been given these complainers to nurse.

> Whence should I have flesh to give unto all this people? for
> they weep unto me, saying, Give us flesh, that we may eat.
> I am not able to bear all this people alone, because *it is* too
> heavy for me.[12]

So God heard the complaint of Moses and allowed the appointment of
helpers to organize and to lead the people. But God was not happy with
the complainers and their whining about meat.

> And I will come down and talk with thee there: and I will
> take of the spirit which *is* upon thee, and will put *it* upon
> them; and they shall bear the burden of the people with thee,
> that thou bear *it* not thyself alone. And say thou unto the
> people, Sanctify yourselves against to morrow, and ye shall
> eat flesh: for ye have wept in the ears of the LORD, saying,
> Who shall give us flesh to eat? for *it was* well with us in
> Egypt: therefore the LORD will give you flesh, and ye shall
> eat. Ye shall not eat one day, nor two days, nor five days,
> neither ten days, nor twenty days; *But* even a whole month,
> until it come out at your nostrils, and it be loathsome unto
> you: because that ye have despised the LORD which *is*
> among you, and have wept before him, saying, Why came we
> forth out of Egypt? And Moses said, The people, among
> whom I *am, are* six hundred thousand footmen; and thou hast
> said, I will give them flesh, that they may eat a whole month.

Shall the flocks and the herds be slain for them, to suffice them? or shall all the fish of the sea be gathered together for them, to suffice them? And the LORD said unto Moses, Is the LORD'S hand waxed short? thou shalt see now whether my word shall come to pass unto thee or not.[13]

The Lord caused a great wind to gather millions of quail from the sea and deposit them upon the Israelites. There were so many that it defies imagination. And as soon as the gluttonous group began to eat the flesh of the birds, they began to get sick. Because they had been used to a healthy diet of manna and their digestive systems could not cope with such huge quantities of meat (animal protein and fat) over a period of one month, they became sick and died.

God's anger was hot against those who distrusted Him to satisfy their needs. Therefore, God demonstrated to them that He was all-sufficient and that He could marshal up any amount of anything that they desired in quantities that they could not even imagine. He also demonstrated that our selfish desires are not healthy and that they lead to sickness and death.

How to Live, How to Eat, How to Worship

This story reveals several important truths to us. First, **God provides daily needs** for His people, but they must trust Him daily. The manna lasted only one day because Jehovah Jirah ("God is our Provider") wanted the people to seek Him every day for sustenance and for guidance. On the day before the Sabbath, the manna would last two days. Even in a place as dry as the desert, God can provide sustenance for the body, if we but trust and obey Him.

Secondly, **God provides a diet of meat not for health but for survival** if no other food is available. God allowed Noah and the rest of humanity to kill animals and eat the flesh thereof for survival in a hostile world where vegetation was in limited supply. The desert had very little vegetation and certainly could not furnish food for such a throng as two million Jews and their livestock. Because they lusted for meat and disregarded God's perfect provision, they suffered the consequences.

Thirdly, **God provided meat for the purpose of showing us that shedding of blood is necessary for the remission of sins**. What better way to preview the sacrifice of His Son, Jesus, than to remind them that at every sin there must be shedding of blood. God demonstrated this in the Garden of Eden when He made clothes for Adam and Eve with the skin of an animal He had killed. God also demonstrated the necessity of eating meat for survival when He commanded that the priests eat part of the sacrifice to show the life it gives to the eater. As Christ's blood and body must be partaken of for survival from sin, so the priest's survival depends on eating the meat of the sin sacrifice.

In the wilderness God guided His people, protected them, provided for them, and trained them in His ways through Moses and the giving of the law. The Levitical Law detailed how the people were to live, to eat, and to worship. In the next chapter we will see how God also taught them that they were privileged to be His dwelling place among the nations.

---

[1] *The Holy Bible : King James Version.*, 1 Sa 15:22. Oak Harbor, WA: Logos Research Systems, Inc., 1995.

[2] *The Holy Bible : King James Version.*, Heb 9:22. Oak Harbor, WA: Logos Research Systems, Inc., 1995.

[3] *The Holy Bible : King James Version.*, Ge 3:21. Oak Harbor, WA: Logos Research Systems, Inc., 1995.

[4] *Logos Hymnal.* 1st edition. Oak Harbor, WA: Logos Research Systems, Inc., 1995.

[5] *The Holy Bible : King James Version.*, Jn 6:53-59. Oak Harbor, WA: Logos Research Systems, Inc., 1995.

[6] *The Holy Bible : King James Version.*, Ex 16:1-5. Oak Harbor, WA: Logos Research Systems, Inc., 1995.

[7] Henry, Matthew. *Matthew Henry's Commentary on the Whole Bible : Complete and Unabridged in One Volume*, Nu 11:4. Peabody: Hendrickson, 1996, c1991.

[8] *The Holy Bible : King James Version.*, Ex 16:13-15. Oak Harbor, WA: Logos Research Systems, Inc., 1995.

[9] *The Holy Bible : King James Version.*, Ex 17:5-6. Oak Harbor, WA: Logos Research Systems, Inc., 1995.

[10] http://www.tidings.org/readings/readings0299.htm

[11] *The Holy Bible : King James Version.*, Le 26:3-13. Oak Harbor, WA: Logos Research Systems, Inc., 1995.

[12] *The Holy Bible : King James Version.*, Nu 11:13-14. Oak Harbor, WA: Logos Research Systems, Inc., 1995.

[13] *The Holy Bible : King James Version.*, Nu 11:17-23. Oak Harbor, WA: Logos Research Systems, Inc., 1995.

CHAPTER 5

THE TABERNACLE OF GOD IS WITH MEN

A People For His Temple

A very unique event occurred in the exodus of the Jews from Egypt. God had previously revealed himself and His ways to His chosen ones through the patriarchs. But when Moses led the Israelites out of the Egyptian captivity, He chose to visibly lead them through the pillar of cloud by day and the pillar of fire by night. These two very visible manifestations were undeniable indications that the Jews were His chosen people and a vessel themselves of His will and way.

When God breathed the breath of life into Adam and he became a living soul (Genesis 2:7), mankind became a dwelling place for the Spirit of God, a tabernacle for the Creator of the universe. Of course, God is omnipresent and is not limited by space or time or a physical body, but nonetheless, He chooses to inhabit His bride, the Church, the body of Christ.

"In the Old Testament, God had a temple for His people; in the New Testament, God has a people for His temple."(Dr. D. James Kennedy) In the Old Testament, God chose to speak through the patriarchs, the priests, and the prophets, as He spoke through them. During the exodus, God spoke through Moses and dwelt in a cloud by day and a pillar of fire by night. He then chose to demonstrate His desire to live in and among His children by dwelling in a tabernacle meticulously constructed and full of rich symbolism. The word tabernacle means tent or covering.

> And let them make me a sanctuary; that I may dwell among
> them. According to all that I shew thee, *after* the pattern of
> the tabernacle, and the pattern of all the instruments thereof,
> even so shall ye make *it*.[1]

In the rich symbolism of the tabernacle instructions, God has shown us how He wants us to house Him. He is worthy of the best of rooms. He is holy and hates sin. He is righteous and spotlessly clean. He is a God of order and cleanliness. He is perfectly righteous. He is God Almighty and must be approached with respect and honor. He is the God of love and mercy, reaching out to sinful man with salvation, forgiveness, and eternal life.

Why did God want Moses to build such a structure? Yes, indeed, He wanted to sanctify His people and set them apart for Godly service in the midst of a heathen world. But more than that, I believe that He wanted to demonstrate that the ultimate temple, or tabernacle, was to be the body, mind, and heart of his adopted child, where His throne is gloriously adorned in majesty. The Apostle Paul in Corinthians and John the Beloved in Revelation said it this way.

> Know ye not that ye are the temple of God, and *that* the Spirit
> of God dwelleth in you? If any man defile the temple of God,
> him shall God destroy; for the temple of God is holy, which
> *temple* ye are.[2]

> And I heard a great voice out of heaven saying, Behold, the
> tabernacle of God *is* with men, and he will dwell with them,
> and they shall be his people, and God himself shall be with
> them, *and be* their God.[3]

If we truly are supposed to be the temple of God Almighty on earth, then how should we care for this temple in a cursed world? The Bible gives us several diets that man has used through the ages and it seems that they have gradually diverged from the Genesis diet. Why is this? Has God changed His mind? And if He has changed His mind, how can Christians reconcile that to the scripture that says that God is never-changing?

> Jesus Christ the same yesterday, and today, and for ever.
> Hebrews 13:8

PERMISSION FOR PALATABLE PASSIONS

God has not changed His mind about perfection. His laws of the universe are still in force. Jump off a high building and you will die. Why is it so hard to believe that a terrible diet can also bring injury and death? What's the difference in praying "Father, please heal me" after jumping off a four story building, and in praying "Father, please heal me" after gorging myself for years on deadly foods? Both consequences are the result of breaking God's laws of physics and chemistry. And yet we pray "We see through a glass darkly" all the while not realizing that we have broken a natural law and must pay the price.

Why are we so surprised that a person who is a fine Christian suddenly dies of a heart attack when that fine Christian has disregarded (mostly out of ignorance, but sometimes out of indifference) the laws of God in regard to proper fuel for his body and regular exercise?. Why do we just say, "It was his time to go" when that person could have lived years longer with vitality if he had just known how to fuel and care for his miraculously-designed temple.

However, it is obvious that God has allowed mankind to "fudge" on the perfect diet. Prior to the flood, there is no record of man eating meat or cooked food. The average lifespan of mankind was over 900 years even after God expelled Adam and Eve from the Garden. Even outside the perfect garden, mankind was able to live long lives because of the perfection of the world that God had made. Yes, killing entered the world after the Fall. Yes, death and evil ruled in the new world after the Fall. But lest we forget, the world still had a canopy of protection about it and the plant and animal kingdoms still flourished even though killing had entered the picture. The animals were still very big and so was man.

The dinosaurs were very much alive and as mentioned in Job, were marvelous and awesome (Job 41).

Post-Deluvian Diet

It wasn't until after the flood, when God decided that He had to let mankind eat animal flesh, that He relaxed the rule on diet for survival's sake. That's when the age span of mankind went from the nine hundreds to less than one hundred and twenty years (Genesis 6). Admittedly, there are some other factors such as increased radiation, reduced gene pool, and changes in atmospheric pressure and gases, but these are factors that we cannot change. Diet, on the other hand, is something that is available to us, though we are not able to perfectly duplicate the Garden of Eden diet.

So what is it about this new diet that caused such a drastic change in health? If diet is the only way Christians can return to the Garden of Eden health, what is the role of animals in our new environment? How can we better fuel our body temples and allow them to heal themselves in this day and age? The answer to those questions has been argued back and forth for decades. I'm afraid that the church has failed in answering those questions because it has disregarded the original perfect plan of God in fueling our miraculous self-healing bodies.

Dangerous Animal Foods

Animal flesh, raw or cooked, is void of fiber, the "broom" that cleans our digestive tract of undigested and poisonous leftovers. Cellulose fiber is abundant in raw fruits, vegetables, nuts, and seeds. There is no argument among scientists that fiber is vital for health. There is **NO fiber** in wild animal flesh, or livestock such as beef, chicken, lamb, swine, fowl, or fish. **Zero.**

Animal flesh contains cholesterol, which clogs the arteries of those who eat it, causing cardiovascular disease, CVD. Plants have **NO CHOLESTEROL**. As if mankind had not been told about a menu for health, modern physicians are just realizing that the Bible diet from Genesis is the only diet that can arrest and reverse cardiovascular disease. **A study by one of America's most widely-respected**

surgeons, Dr. Caldwell Esselstyne, has revealed that this disease can be halted and reversed by the plant-based diet. As stated by Dr. Esselstyne, the cultures that depend solely on plant-based nutrition are the healthiest.

> However, coronary artery disease is virtually absent in cultures that eat plant-based diets, such as the Tarahumara Indians of northern Mexico, the Papua highlanders of New Guinea, and the inhabitants of rural China and central Africa. Hundreds of thousands of rural Chinese go for years without a single documented myocardial infarction.[4]

Dr. Esselstyn's twelve-year study is documented on his web site at www.heartattackproof.com. The participants in his study did not have one cardiac event in the 12 years of the study while on the plant-based diet.

Another dangerous ingredient in animal flesh is its protein. In the book titled "The China Study", world renowned biochemist T. Colin Campbell has documented research that has pointed to animal protein as a carcinogen that promotes the growth of cancer cells. That's right. Numerous research has shown that animal protein promotes the growth of cancer while plant foods deter, stop, and even reverse the growth of cancer. The China Study is the largest study ever attempted that compares diet and lifestyle to health. This monumental study performed over 300 tests on thousands of Chinese in distinct people groups. A perfect laboratory, where one people group stay in their home areas all their lives and live off the same diet the entire lifespan, this study pointed out that with only small additions of animal flesh in the diet, degenerative diseases entered into the population. Where no animal flesh was included, there was no occurrence of heart disease, cancer, diabetes, and other degenerative diseases.[5]

Raw flesh is inherently dangerous because it has no natural packaging and it normally contains harmful bacteria, especially in the intestines. Because many people have died from harmful bacteria contained in contaminated meats, the nation and the World Health Organization has become enamored with irradiation. Irradiation is the modern version of pasteurization, but instead of boiling a liquid to kill bacteria, the food is radiated by powerful particles to kill E.coli O157:H7 and Salmonella, two of the deadliest bacteria known. According to the Center for Disease Control on their questions and answers page dealing with food irradiation, the major government agencies have all given approval to food irradiation, not only meats, but fruits and vegetables, as well as other packaged foods. The CDC puts their stamp of approval on this new processing method for giving food long shelf life and safety from contamination.[6]

As I understand it, when our food is irradiated, the particles will kill any live organism in the food, including beneficial bacteria, live enzymes, and will cause the production of lots of free radicals, which live food is famous for fighting. Thanks to our appetite for flesh, we will get little live benefit from our food supply and much more free radical damage to our bodies unless we depend on organic, non-radiated foods.

Animal flesh is also void of the nutrients that are abundant in raw plant foods. Some of these nutrients are phytochemicals, carotenoids, flavenoids, and live enzymes. Almost daily, scientists are discovering new chemicals contained in raw foods that have great beneficial effect on the body. When we eat flesh products, we are eliminating that wonderful synergy of God-given chemicals that help our body to remain healthy.

The most dangerous ingredient of meat products nowadays is the almost certain prospect of contamination by prions, mutated proteins that are the cause of Creutzfeldt - Jakob disease, which is Mad Cow Disease in humans. Called bovine spongiform encephalopathy or BSE for short, this disease is named because of its effect on the brain of cows. It is characterized by the spongy brain that results when the prions eat holes in the brain of the infected animal. CJD, the human strain of the disease, is almost indistinguishable from Parkinson's disease. Our inspection process of meats is woefully inadequate to detect Mad Cow Disease in America's livestock. BSE is so virulent that pathologists are reluctant to undertake an autopsy because they risk contracting it. Autopsy is at present the only way to determine whether the animal has the disease. BSE is believed to have a 10 to 30-year incubation period, therefore organically-fed animals may still have the prions.

The man who woke the nation up to the dangers of ruminant fed beef - that is, beef that are fed flesh from cows, horses, sheep, goats, etc. – was a Montana cowboy named Howard Lyman. He and Oprah Winfrey were sued by the cattle industry for their comments on national television about the dangers of eating beef. But they won their lawsuit in 1998 and Mr. Lyman has gone on to write a book, Mad Cowboy, detailing the history of Mad Cow Disease and the practices of our beef industry that could lead to millions dying of this incurable disease, which literally eats holes in the brain.[7]

I believe that God's natural law has been violated among the animal kingdom. Animals were originally created to eat plants. When sin entered the world, animals began eating animals. **When livestock growers began feeding dead animal parts to live animals, the diseases began to increase and now we are at a critical stage when millions of humans could be infected with this deadly, incurable, wasting disease.**

With all this information detailing the danger and unhealthiness of animal products, why do we insist on defiling our body-temples by eating animal products? In my opinion, there are a number of reasons:

Adamant Addiction to Animals

Some deny the mounting evidence that animal products are bad for health. Many doubt that God would allow an animal diet to be harmful. There is the social pressure to conform to what others are eating. Others have a disdain for those who have the discipline of a plant-based diet. Many suffer from disillusionment brought on by conflicting information from government, industry, medical, and scientific communities. There are also those who are disinterested and just float along with the herd. I'm sure there are some who just want to be disobedient to any kind of authority. Lastly, most medical doctors are not trained in nutrition and are useless in educating people to the dangers of animal products. Whatever the reason, most are suffering from an addiction to animal products that is real and painful at times of denial. And probably all suffer from being a victim of convenience, because organic, raw, nutritious, delicious, convenient, fast foods are often hard to find and more expensive.

I believe that the main reason people insist on eating animal products is that we are all gluttons by nature. We are all sinners by choice and by birth. We desire that which is good-tasting, beautiful, easily-obtained, and cheap. Fasting is foreign to most of us. Eating just exactly what we want, when we want it, and in "value sized" portions is our daily fare. After all, what was the original sin? Disregarding God's wise instruction about what to eat, resulting in gluttony and death.

---

[1] *The Holy Bible : King James Version.*, Ex 25:7-9. Oak Harbor, WA: Logos Research Systems, Inc., 1995.

[2] *The Holy Bible : King James Version.*, I Corinthians 3:16. Oak Harbor, WA: Logos Research Systems, Inc., 1995.

[3] The Holy Bible : King James Version., Revelation 21:3. Oak Harbor, WA: Logos Research Systems, Inc., 1995.

[4] http://heartattackproof.com/resolving_cade.htm.

[5] Campbell, T. Colin. The China Study (Dallas: Benbella Books, 2005).

[6] http://www.cdc.gov/ncidod/dbmd/diseaseinfo/foodirradiation.htm

[7] Lyman, Howard F. Mad Cowboy (New York: Simon & Schuster, 1998).

CHAPTER 6

TRANSITION FROM OMNIVOROUS TO HERBIVOROUS

ADMISSIONS OF AN ANIMAL ADDICT

Up until a few years ago, I never really considered fasting. I was raised on meat at every meal. I ate bacon, eggs, and/or sausage for breakfast every day. I ate chicken, calf liver, roast, shrimp, and catfish almost every week for lunch and supper. If my mother had not also included peas, sweet potatoes, corn, butter beans, squash, okra, snap beans, bananas, apples, oranges, and tomatoes in our daily diet, I probably would have died of cancer, heart disease, or some other degenerative disease years ago.

My parents obviously suffered physically for their diet, because both of them died of heart disease. My grandfather died of Parkinson's disease and my grandmother died of heart disease. I must have inherited some strong genes from my dad's mom, who lived to be ninety-five. I was born sick and had to have a blood transfusion from my mom. Rheumatic fever afflicted me at age six, leaving me with an enlarged heart and a heart murmur, which kept me out of the Viet Nam War. Regular sinus infections and the frequent use of over-the-counter drugs and prescription antibiotics probably weakened my liver and pancreas.

CONFESSIONS OF A CONFECTIONER

My favorite drink was Dr. Pepper. I was almost as much a "pepper" as was portrayed by Forrest Gump in the movie by the same name. We normally bought five pounds of processed sugar every other week and more during the holidays. I remember my mom would make cakes during the Christmas holiday season. Our favorite was caramel squares, loaded with eggs, white flour, and pure white sugar, caramelized into a golden icing. It's a wonder we ever made it to adulthood! But those were special occasions, and we didn't eat that kind of food daily as a lot of folks do today.

It is amazing how we all have become sugar addicts. When I compare my past experiences with sugar eating and the habits of today's children, teenagers, and adults, I see that there is a definite increase in our sugar consumption, for it is in virtually every food. Nowadays, instead of cane sugar ingredients, it is in the form of beet sugar or corn sugar. Try to find a processed food that doesn't have some corn sugar in it and you will be hard-pressed. The USDA Economic Research Service, one of fourteen USDA service agencies, says, "The United States is the largest consumer of sweeteners, including high fructose corn syrup, and is one of the largest global sugar importers."[1]

Processed sugar is a contributing factor to many diseases as listed by Nancy Appleton, PhD, in her book, Lick the Sugar Habit. In the book she documents clinical evidence of 124 ways that sugar ruins your health. Some of those include suppressing the immune system, upsetting the mineral relationships in the body, causing a significant rise in triglycerides, reducing high-density lipoproteins, interfering with the absorption of calcium and magnesium, and causing tooth decay, asthma, and arthritis.[2]

THE GREAT AWAKENING

About the mid 90s I began to rethink my diet and lifestyle. Did the Lord really mean that our body was to be a temple not only free of drugs and alcohol, but also of dangerous foods as well? Could my diet have been destructive all throughout my life without me realizing it? More and more evidence was put in front of me, and I began to understand that the original diet was the only way to health and longevity.

In my calling as a Minister of Music in Southern Baptist churches I was caught up in the lifestyle that has led to the demise of many good men and women in the ministry. That lifestyle was full of meat and dairy products, sugary desserts, salt, candy, carbonated beverages, snacks loaded with dangerous additives, and a habit of no exercise except on rare occasions. Year after year, I battled sinus infections that were the scourge of singers in the ministry. At least twice a year I was unable to lead worship because of sinus drainage into my larynx causing a deep hoarseness and robbing me of my tenor notes. At least twice a year the doctor would prescribe a powerful round of antibiotics that had little effect on the real cause of my sinus infections. Year after year, I pondered this lifestyle and asked myself, "Is there a better way?"

One Sunday evening, on an occasion when my church was not having evening services, I found myself attending the services of a fellow Minister of Music. He was my mentor in the music ministry. A wonderful servant of the Lord and a great example of dedication to the music ministry, my friend was leading youth choir as I entered the church. I had come too early, so I told him I would wait in the sanctuary until service time. After a few minutes, a youth burst into the sanctuary and said that something had happened to my friend. I ran to the choir room and found him lying flat on the floor, being attended by paramedics. I comforted his wife, who was the accompanist for him, as they carried him down two flights of stairs to the waiting ambulance. Several times they sought to restore sinus rhythm to his heart - but to no avail. I followed the ambulance to the emergency room where I talked with the EMT's about his condition. They told me in tears that they could not get him to revive. I comforted them and later met with the Pastor as he prayed with my friend's wife. The funeral of this dear brother in the faith was one of the most wonderful worship services I have ever experienced. Our state's Minister of Music chorus sang from the choir and great music was offered up in praise of our Savior and for this great servant who had fallen in combat.

Later I pondered on why I was at that church on that particular day. It was a Sunday, when 99% of the time I would be at my church leading choir and worship. But this day I was at my friend's church. Why? Could God be telling me something? It sure seemed like it. So I began thinking and praying for the answer. My friend had suffered for years

with high blood pressure, being overweight, and with little exercise.
Many of my friends in the ministry were like him, and I was right along
there with them. Could God be calling me to change my lifestyle and
to warn my friends in the ministry?

The final exclamation point was added when my wife, Marilyn,
experienced several years of suffering, first with endometriosis
followed by an endoscopic hysterectomy and then fibromyalgia. Nine
medical doctors and numerous diagnoses failed to get at the problem
that caused her pain. One night she hurt so much that she actually
planned her funeral in tears. The Lord heard our cries for help and a
friend brought us news about the Hallelujah Diet®[3]. It was a plant based
diet of 85% raw food, 15% cooked food, lots of fresh carrot juice, a
dehydrated barley powder, and distilled water. We watched a two-hour
video from a preacher who had been cured of colon cancer by following
the diet. It was very similar to God's original diet in Genesis 1:29
because it eliminated all animal products and processed foods. We
agreed to try it for a few weeks. After three months she was no better
and she asked me if we could quit it. I told her we ought to try it a few
more weeks. **Three weeks later she told me that she felt no
symptoms of the disease!**

Cautiously we kept with the diet and week after week it brought better
health and fewer sick days. We learned to rethink our eating habits and
our grocery buying habits. We threw away boxes and boxes of
processed foods and restocked with fresh produce and lots of carrots
and spinach. Meat was no longer in our freezer, our refrigerator, or on
our table. Milk was replaced with distilled water and rice milk.
Walking, jogging, running, and lifting weights were now a daily part of
our lives. My regular bouts with sinusitis and infections were gone. We
threw away ALL our prescription drugs and even the over-the-counter
drugs, including aspirin, Tylenol, cough medicines and sinus medicines.
We were now drug-free, and disease-free! As I write this, it has been
seven years since we have had the illnesses that regularly affected us.
We are not on a diet anymore but a lifestyle of health and wellness.

> Praise to the Lord, who with marvelous wisdom hath made thee,
> Decked thee with health and with loving hand guided and stayed thee!
> How oft in grief
> Hath not He brought thee relief,
> Spreading His wings for to shade thee![4]

The scriptures about our body temples began to come alive and take on new meaning for us. We realized anew that the Bible can be interpreted literally far more than we had first believed. Our body temples should be cared for just as the first tabernacle had been cared for. The diet discipline we have now brings honor to our Lord, who is glorified by our healthy, vibrant lives. The time spent now in Bible reading, writing, worship, and witnessing is not robbed by illness, drugs, surgery, and slavery to eating. **We have no fear of cancer, heart disease, or spending our last days in a rest home. Fasting is a regular part of our lives, strengthening our discipline in other areas as well as in the physical.**

> Bless the LORD, O my soul: and all that is within me, *bless* his holy name. Bless the LORD, O my soul, and forget not all his benefits: Who forgiveth all thine iniquities; who healeth all thy diseases; Who redeemeth thy life from destruction; who crowneth thee with lovingkindness and tender mercies; Who satisfieth thy mouth with good *things; so that* thy youth is renewed like the eagle's.[5]

My calling is now clear - I believe that God has called me to awaken the sleeping church to a healthier, and more effective ministry that can lengthen our term of service here on earth and win this battle for the body of the saints.

---

[1] http://www.ers.usda.gov/Briefing/Sugar/

[2] Lick the Sugar Habit, Appleton, Nancy, PhD. Avery, Santa Monica, CA, 1996.

[3] God's Way to Ultimate Health. Malkmus, George. (Hallelujah Acres Publishing, Shelby, N.C.) 1995.

[4] *Praise to the Lord the Almighty*, Joachim Neander. Logos Hymnal. 1st edition. Oak Harbor, WA: Logos Research Systems, Inc., 1995.

[5] The Holy Bible : King James Version., Ps 103:1-5. Oak Harbor, WA: Logos Research Systems, Inc., 1995.

CHAPTER 7

OLD TESTIMENT TEMPLE PARALLELS

IDOLS IN OUR TEMPLES

In II Kings 21:7 and in II Chronicles 33:3 we are told that King Manasseh made and put into the temple idols that desecrated the temple of Jehovah. As the Southern Kingdom progressed more and more toward destruction and captivity, so waned the presence of the Spirit of God in His temple. After the captivity of Judah in Babylon, the prophet Ezekiel was shown in a vision the process of desecration of the temple and the priests as recorded in Ezekiel 8.

> He said also unto me, Turn thee yet again, *and* thou shalt see greater abominations that they do. Then he brought me to the door of the gate of the LORD'S house which *was* toward the north; and, behold, there sat women weeping for Tammuz.[1]

As I read Matthew Henry's commentary on this passage, I was struck by the similarities then and now. Tammuz, one of the idols of the Assyrians, was mourned because he died. This passage showed that one of the four sins of the desecrated temple was shown to be an idol of death. This idol of Judah can be compared to the idols of our day.

An abominable thing indeed that any should choose rather to
serve an idol in tears than to serve the true God *with
joyfulness and gladness of heart!* [2]

What idols are keeping us from the Lord of Lords? Could it be that we
are trusting in drugs and doctors more than in the Living God and His
perfect diet? How my heart breaks each time I hear of a saint who has
resolved to follow the doctor's orders and submit to deadly radiation,
chemotherapy, and surgery or to a life of dangerous drugs and prison in
rest homes! **How discouraging it is to a Health Minister for fellow
brothers and sisters in Christ to be totally oblivious to the highly
probable deliverance from disease waiting for the disciplined return
to God's original diet and lifestyle!. What a shame it is for a soldier
of the cross to give up the fight for life because of a lack of faith in
the miraculous self-healing body given to us by the Master
Designer.**

Amazing Lack of Faith

It amazes me that people can be so blind to the true God of healing.
Instead of trusting in the healing power of our divinely-designed,
miraculously self- healing bodies, we rely on invasive, destructive, and
ineffective means which cost thousands and thousands of dollars.

It amazes me that brilliant medical doctors can be so intelligent yet so
blind to the true way of healing. Blindly, most M.D.'s ignore the root
cause of a cancer and mechanically prescribe treatment that doesn't
remotely address the cause of the problem. Why is it that the widely-
recognized causes of cancer are totally ignored when treatment options
are given? Those causes are so obvious! Is it just a coincidence that
people groups who eat a plant-based diet have no cancer at all? **The
China Project** [3] **has provided real evidence that cancer is brought
on by animal products in the diet. Heart disease is a result of eating
animal products as proven by the Esselstyn** [4] **study and many
others.** Osteoporosis and breast cancer are unknown to people who eat
a plant- based diet.

Could it be that we are in denial of the true cause of our problems when
we consent to having our organs cut out and our body mutilated than to
change our diet and lifestyle, letting God's wonderful healing take

place naturally when we fast from dangerous foods? Does surgery cure cancer? The American Cancer Society lists eight reasons why surgery is used for cancer treatment. Preventative surgery is done even when the cancer is NON-MALIGNANT. Diagnostic surgery is done to determine IF there is cancer. Staging surgery is done to determine the EXTENT of the cancer. Curative (misnomer) surgery is done in hopes of removing ALL of the cancer. Debulking (Cytoreductive) surgery is done when they think that they CAN'T remove all of it. Palliative surgery is done to treat COMPLICATIONS of cancer. Supportive surgery is sometimes needed to ENABLE other cancer treatments. And lastly, Restorative surgery is necessary when other surgeries have to be TIDIED up.[5] NONE of these reasons address the cause of the cancer, nor guarantee that it will not return. This list does not include other approaches that attempt to diagnose, burn, freeze, or electrocute cancer. **Is this not a god that is worshipped instead of the true God of healing?**

Every effect has a cause. Cancer is not caused by a lack of surgery or radiation or chemo. Something causes cancer. I believe that cancer is caused by what we eat and drink. It is a natural law that when we abuse our body and give it junk, cancer is a real probability. I don't even have to document that fact, it is so widely accepted. Then why is it so widely denied that to remedy that consequence we must change our eating habits? Many would rather spend millions of dollars on health insurance, surgery, chemo, radiation, dangerous drugs, and then give to cancer charities, which do little to promote the real cure for cancer. It seems that we want to keep our gluttonous lifestyles and spend our fortunes on pills, surgery, radiation, chemo, and, more recently, gene altering, to avoid the discipline of healthy living. **The Israelites did the same thing we are doing. They denied the power of God's temple and God left it to destruction because they ran after other gods of pleasure and convenience.**

There are many wonderful medical doctors out there ~~would~~ *that* would love to teach preventive health care but are chained to the protocol that the medical schools and state medical boards have taught them. The American Medical Association studied research after research and came to the conclusions that a plant-based diet is the diet that offers the best protection from coronary heart disease, CHD.

ᴧ wow !

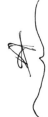

Conclusions Substantial evidence indicates that diets using non-hydrogenated unsaturated fats as the predominant form of dietary fat, whole grains as the main form of carbohydrates, an abundance of fruits and vegetables, and adequate omega-3 fatty acids can offer significant protection against CHD. Such diets, together with regular physical activity, avoidance of smoking, and maintenance of a healthy body weight, may prevent the majority of cardiovascular disease in Western populations. [6]

Our medical community has sold itself out to the drug companies in search of riches to the detriment of true healing by prevention. Dr. John McDougall, for over 30 years a proponent of the vegan lifestyle through his books, clinic, and T.V., has summarized the problem in his newsletter, Star McDougallers, on his web site, www.drmcdougall.com.

One of the most common questions I am asked is; why don't other doctors practice diet-therapy? Here are a few things I have noticed:

1) Diet-therapy is not paid for by insurance companies, so this makes it hard for doctors to have a financially successful practice—their family has to eat too.

2) Diet-therapy is not a respected field of medical research or practice. Revered scientists study genetics, biochemistry, virology and pharmacology. Surgeons and specialists are considered next-to-God talented in their practices. After all, how smart do you have to be to tell someone to eat beans and rice to cure heart disease?

3) The patient adds an extra variable to medical care in diet-therapy—they have to perform the treatment. With surgery all a doctor has to do is cut them open, and an Internist only has to have them swallow a pill.

4) You have to walk the talk. A doctor prescribing a healthy diet and exercise must do both. Steak and cheesecake, and similar fare, are still served at every noontime hospital conference and Heart Association meeting.

5) *Diet-therapy is not "the community standard of practice."*
In a malpractice suit you are judged by this standard, and if
you practice like other doctors, even if the patient dies, you are
on the right side of the law.

6) *Doctors never learn to make referrals to diet-therapy—they*
refer to the specialist, including the psychiatrist, but rarely the
dietitian.

7) *In medical school today, training students receive*
essentially no education on diet-therapy.

8) *A very few doctors may realize that diet-therapy is*
counterproductive—if the patients became well, they would no
longer be patients. Those running the pharmaceutical
companies, however, do realize the danger of the public
becoming aware of the true potential of diet vs. drugs—so they
fund research and place advertisements that directly attack the
truth.

The bottom line is to not expect help from your doctor on
matters of chronic disease, but instead to learn about the
benefits of a low-fat vegan diet, exercise, and clean habits and
free yourself of the medical businesses.[7]

There are some doctors that do teach diet-therapy. And praise God for
them! They recognize that the education they have been given is
flawed. The medical schools have not taught them nutrition and
preventive healing. The training they have received only covers
symptoms and hardly ever addresses the root causes of disease, which
is diet and lifestyle. May their numbers increase!

I know many good Christian doctors who realize that drugs and surgery
are not the best way to health, but are chained to the peer review
protocols that the medical boards prescribe. Many a fine doctor would
love to be able to use diet and lifestyle to help his/her patients if they
would not have their licenses revoked. Of course they would have to
read the scientific journals and bone up on natural nutrition before they
could be helpful.

Hallelujah Acres has a list of hundreds of testimonies of people who have been healed of virtually every disease known to man by simply changing their diet and lifestyle. One of the best of these testimonies comes from an OB-GYN doctor who discovered by needle biopsy he had prostate cancer. He decided to go the Hallelujah Diet way and to fast from meats, dairy, sugar, bleached flour products, table salt, and processed foods. He began to juice carrots and other vegetables and to jog daily. Six months later he had another biopsy that showed no cancer cells. His cancer doctor, thinking that he had missed the cancer cells ordered eighteen needle biopsies. None showed any signs of cancer! This doctor now tells others about the plant-based diet that can allow the body to heal itself of cancer. This type of testimony has been repeated hundreds of times. The web site where these testimonies are cataloged and listed is www.hacres.com.

The most difficult diseases to reverse are the ones that are very advanced, but even those can be helped and be brought under control when the diet and lifestyle are changed drastically and with determination. As recorded in the Bible's chronology of the Southern Kingdom, the dramatic revivals from bad kings to good kings is breathtaking. When the Israelites returned to God, He forgave and healed them. It is the same with our bodies. These miraculous bodies can heal themselves when with faith and discipline we fuel them with the foods that they were designed to have.

As we study the decline of the temple in the Old Testament, it is obvious that when God's house is neglected, He eventually leaves it. As the divided kingdoms continued to deteriorate, so did the temple. Finally, God's glory left the temple desolate. I'm afraid that is what has happened to many Christians. We have let into our temples foods and beverages and chemicals that are idols to us. We revere our cheeseburgers, hot dogs, carbonated beverages, chicken fingers, barbeque, roast beef, sweet tea, steaks, ice cream, and cake, as well as personal care items that load our body down with toxins. Most of us are addicted to television as couch potatoes. Christians spend much of their time at church feasting and playing, but very little time fasting and praying. We may be disciplined in Bible study and prayer but sadly lacking in body disciplines like fasting, exercise, healthy eating, and rest. It's as though we have accepted Jesus as Lord of our souls but not Lord of our appetites. It is time to clean up our temples!

WORSHIP OF FOREIGN GODS

Now this may be a stretch, but in some respects Christians have
worshipped foreign gods when we elevate our medical doctor to the
position of our authority in matters of health. It should be innocent
enough to seek professional advice in regard to a health problem. But
the professionals we put on pedestals are sometimes not qualified to
give us the best advice about physical health. In a survey of medical
student seniors by the American Association of Medical Colleges, the
students as well as the practicing physicians were asked to judge
whether their "Nutrition-related experiences were adequate". 44.7% of
the students disagreed with this statement. Likewise, the Intersociety
Professional Nutritional Education Consortium has this to say about
physician competency in nutrition.

> Given the prevalence of nutritionally-related chronic diseases
> in American society, the training of physicians should include
> a focus on the relationships of diet to disease. Yet, in spite of
> scientific data, public interest, U.S. government reports,
> society studies, and congressional mandates, the teaching of
> nutrition in medical schools and residency programs remains
> inadequate. Physicians thus remain insufficiently informed
> about the role of diet in the prevention and treatment of
> disease. [8]

 Many times I have heard the doctor quoted as saying, when asked if diet
could help a disease, "It doesn't matter. Eat anything you want. It's a
matter of genetics." What foolishness! What ignorance! What a
copout! And most of us blindly follow his or her advice to take
dangerous medication that only masks the symptoms and does nothing
to address the cause of the malady. **We have elevated these
professionals to such heights that we don't even question them. And
in many instances they degrade a nutritionally-educated
practitioner who has proper education to deliver the patient back
to health.**

According to the Center for Disease Control, five of the ten leading
causes of death in the United States are attributed to diet and lifestyle. [9]
And yet, our trained physicians have little more than a beginner course
in nutrition. In some regards, we have substituted an idol for the living

God. Instead of God's original perfect plan for health, we substitute the advice of a "professional" who is often ignorant about the latest scientific facts of nutrition.

Now that I have turned most doctors against me, let me say that it's not entirely their fault. Who trains them? The scientists supported by the government and drug companies, of course. The major contributors of medical schools are the National Institutes of Health, the state legislatures and the drug companies. Do you believe that these entities are going to promote nutritional training for physicians and thus eliminate the need for drug and treatment research? Of course not! The medical schools get billions of dollars of tax money for carrying on the research that almost totally ignores nutritional research. Only public opinion will force them to do that.

We must wake up to the brain-washing that our medical schools have dished out to our finest students. Let us encourage them to get additional training in nutrition and to use experienced and well-trained practitioners to help their patients learn true nutritional information. **When our doctors begin to practice preventive medicine instead of drug prescriptions, then our nation's health will return to the place it should be. Then and only then will we turn back the tide of temple desolation for Christians.**

One of the most refreshing articles I have read details how a medical student, Michael Mantz, interned with Dr. Joel Fuhrman, author of Eat to Live. Having spent a year interning with doctors who utilized conventional care, the contrast was stark when he spent a few months with Dr. Fuhrman.

> "Patients would come in and out in less than 15 minutes and they usually were prescribed several pharmaceutical drugs to mask/cover up their symptoms. Patients from these doctors never recovered their health because the causes of their problems were never addressed. The underlying theme was always that their patients were genetically-damaged goods who needed to be on drugs for the rest of their lives...In one day at Dr. Fuhrman's office I see many patients who routinely dramatically lower their cholesterol...He prescribed to each of them a class of powerful cholesterol-

lowering substances: fruits, (especially berries) vegetables (especially green ones), beans, and certain nuts and seeds. Dr. Fuhrman helped them with their menu planning and even gave them recipes to make a gourmet meal. I learned about the natural cholesterol-lowering compounds in these natural foods, and which foods had the most potent cholesterol-lowering ability. He made sure each patient did regular exercise commensurate with their ability and lifestyle...The results were astounding. Astounding because every patient we saw achieved similar dramatic improvements."[10]

This is the kind of doctor we need more of. Let me say that I highly respect the doctors who have sacrificed and worked hard because they have a compassion for the sick and a deep calling to restore them to health. I urge them to return to their first love, and that is healing the sick, not covering up the illness. I have no respect, however, for the physician who pads his pocketbook and builds his mansion on earth at the expense of the lives of his patients who are desperately looking to him for help. We need doctors who are trained not only in physiology, diagnosing illness, trauma, and limited medication, but who are also trained in preventive nutrition and healthy lifestyle.

Another problem is the state medical boards that set acceptable medical practice for doctors. These boards frequently punish doctors who choose to use alternative treatments and preventive therapies instead of the traditional ones in their practice. One organization that has arisen to champion the rights of citizens to choose their health practitioners is the Institute for Health Freedom. At their website I found this quote from a medical doctor who is a member of one such licensing board.

Many good doctors with advanced degrees are unwilling to provide complementary therapies because of FDA and local medical society pressures. Despite overwhelming evidence that many complementary therapies are more effective and less costly, many doctors are unwilling to incorporate them into their own practices. **Every doctor practicing Food medicine should be able to incorporate complementary therapies into his or her own practice without fear of retribution from FDA and state medical boards.** (bolding by editor)[11]

The elevation of state medical boards above the free choice of doctors and patients is tantamount to worship of these powerful lawmakers. Until doctors regain their freedom in choosing alternative natural therapies, the trend toward useless, destructive, and expensive medical treatment will continue.

America is like the frog in the kettle. Christians have been lulled into the lukewarm water of over-the-counter drugs and stimulants. The water has become hotter and hotter as we yield to drugs, surgery, radiation, and chemotherapy. Finally, the water is boiling and we just go right along and give up our entire fortunes as we battle a deadly disease without even considering jumping out of the pot and into the green grass of live food and healing.

---

[1] The Holy Bible: King James Version., Ezekiel 8:13-14. Oak Harbor, WA: Logos Research Systems, Inc., 1995.

[2] Henry, Matthew. Matthew Henry's Commentary on the Whole Bible: Complete and Unabridged in One Volume, Ezekiel 8:13. Peabody: Hendrickson, 1996, c1991.

[3] http://www.vegsource.com/event/campbell.htm

[4] http://www.vegsource.com/esselstyn/

[5] http://www.cancer.org/docroot/ETO/content/ETO_1_2X_Surgery.asp#C2

[6] JAMA — Abstract Optimal Diets for Prevention of Coronary Heart Disease, November 27, 2002, Hu and Willett 288 (20) 2569.htm

[7] Star McDougaller. http://www.drmcdougall.com/misc/2006star/060100starralph.htm.

[8] http://main.uab.edu/ipnec/show.asp?durki=35204

[9] http://www.cdc.gov/nccdphp/factsheets/death_causes2000.htm

[10] http://drfuhrman.com/library/article14.aspx

[11] http://www.forhealthfreedom.org/Publications/Monopoly/Born.html

CHAPTER 8

HEATHEN HERESY LEFT AND RIGHT

A New Heresy

There is a new heresy among us that has quietly corrupted our doctrine. Traditionally, heresy is a self-chosen doctrinal departure from God's original plan. Today we call political candidates liberal, moderate, or conservative, left wing, moderate, or right wing. I believe that Christians have been lulled into a departure from the central theme of the Gospel - that is, faith in the Lord Jesus Christ, demonstrated by a sacrificial life, complete with spirit, soul, mind, and body dedicated to Him. There are heretics on the left side of the Gospel who believe that a legalistic approach to Christian living by observing man-made rules and denying fleshly desires will bring salvation and heaven. Then on the right side there exists a spiritualistic approach of free grace and a total disregard for the discipline of the flesh. Neither of these heresies is central to the Gospel where there is love for the Lord with all the soul, spirit, and body. In the New Testament the left-hand heresy was asceticism and the right-hand heresy was a form of Epicureanism. Both were condemned by the Lord Jesus and by the apostle Paul.

Abusive Asceticism — Living Sacrifice — Neoepicureanism

Abusive Asceticism

Asceticism is defined by Nave's Topical Bible as "A philosophy that leads to severe austerities in subordinating the body to the control of the moral attributes of the mind".

> During the fourth century, hundreds of ascetics sought to escape temptation and punish their bodies by living as hermits. The extremes to which they went in their attempts to deny gratification of "physical lusts" seem incredible.
>
> St. Ascepsimas wore so many chains that he had to crawl around on hands and knees. Besarion, a monk, would not even give in to his body's desire for restful sleep—for forty years he would not lie down while sleeping. Macarius the Younger sat naked in a swamp for six months until mosquito bites made him look like a victim of leprosy. St. Maron spent eleven years in a hollowed-out tree trunk. Others lived in caves, dens of beasts, dry wells—even tombs.
>
> To suffer the discomfort of filth, stench, worms, and maggots was considered to be spiritually beneficial and a sign of victory over the body.[1]

This is the sort of apostasy that Paul was speaking of in I Timothy 4:3 when he warned that in the latter days a form of asceticism would seek to deny the freedom that the gospel had brought - that freedom to marry and to eat meat. Yes, Christians are free to marry and to eat meat, even though they are not the ideal for disciplined Christian living. **These freedoms should not be made a test of spirituality.**

PREVIEW PICTURES FROM GOD

In I Timothy 4:3 and in I Corinthians 7:1-2, I believe that the apostle Paul is trying to tell us that meat-eating is sent from God to be a picture of our survival available through Christ Jesus and should not be looked upon as a sin. The same can be said of earthly marriage. It is a picture of our eventual marriage to the Lamb of God.

> Forbidding to marry, *and commanding* to abstain from meats, which God hath created to be received with thanksgiving of them which believe and know the truth.[2]

I believe that God gave us animals to eat for several reasons. **Meat-eating is not the perfect diet. But it is a way to satisfy the powerful hunger of mankind when raw fruits, vegetables, nuts, and seeds are not abundant. It is a way of survival when crops fail and rains don't come. Meat-eating is also used by God to picture how the blood and body of our Lord are to be the only foods for life with Christ.** Animal flesh is allowed by God but is not the perfect diet. Why would God say in Isaiah that the perfect kingdom to come would be one where the wolf would dwell in peace with the lamb? Peace among the animals and peace between animals and mankind - that is the perfection that God intended, not killing and eating of flesh, but nourishment from the plant kingdom.

> The wolf also shall dwell with the lamb, and the leopard shall lie down with the kid; and the calf and the young lion and the fatling together; and a little child shall lead them. And the cow and the bear shall feed; their young ones shall lie down together: and the lion shall eat straw like the ox. And the sucking child shall play on the hole of the asp, and the weaned child shall put his hand on the cockatrice' den. They shall not hurt nor destroy in all my holy mountain: for the earth shall be full of the knowledge of the LORD, as the waters cover the sea.[3]

As for marriage, Paul explains why earthly marriage is a necessary institution in light of the condition of our sinful hearts.

> Now concerning the things whereof ye wrote unto me: *It is* good for a man not to touch a woman. Nevertheless, *to avoid* fornication, let every man have his own wife, and let every woman have her own husband.[4]

In this passage in I Corinthians, Paul admitted that marriage, though instituted by God, was a permissive institution and not a perfect one, since mankind's sinful nature exposed him to lust after sex. So marriage was allowed as a way to satisfy the need for sex with God's approval. Next to the desire for air, water, and food, the desire for sex is very powerful in both men and women. The Lord used marriage to perpetuate mankind and to give us a picture of the intimacy that would one day exist between a Christian and his Lord. Jesus used marriage as a picture of the relationship between mankind and his Creator and between Jesus and the church. Marriage was given to us until the day when Christians will all be married to the Lamb and will no longer be the betrothed of Christ, but the bride of our Lord.

This is my Father's world,
O let me ne'er forget
That though the wrong seems oft so strong,
God is the Ruler yet.
This is my Father's world,
The battle is not done;
Jesus who died shall be satisfied,
And earth and heaven be one.[5]

THE NEW EPICUREANISM

The opposite heresy of asceticism is a modern form of Epicureanism. The Epicureanism of Paul's time was a philosophy which taught that sense perception was the only basis for knowledge and those who followed this heresy were attacked as being atheists. Whereas the original Epicureans found contentment in limiting desires and in the joys and solaces of friendship, the modern sense of Epicureanism is that those who are epicures are lovers of eating and drinking. The early Epicureans were devoted to serene detachment and living a peaceful life with no hope of eternal life. **The more modern version of this heresy seems to be that Christians have, through grace, a license to let our lust for food and beverages run wild, while we preach against sins of sexual promiscuity. Heard any sermons on gluttony lately?**

When I was a boy, my father took me to his slaughterhouse one day. My father was a multi-talented man who was at one time a banker, another time an electrician, still another time a grocer and a butcher. It was as a butcher that he took me to his slaughterhouse that he had built in the woods and I got my first glimpse into how we get our hamburgers and hot dogs and steaks. He even let me shoot one of the cows that he was slaughtering that day. I will never forget the fear that the cow showed as it was led into the chute. Cows are pretty dumb, but I believe that cow knew he was going to die because he put up quite a fuss before he was killed. The smell of blood and death was strong and the cow could sense it perfectly. I never ate another bite of meat that I didn't think about the cow or horse or chicken that gave its life for that morsel of meat.

Today's generation of adults, teenagers, and children have never experienced the slaughter house or the hog-killing. They are oblivious to the pain and fright that animals have before they are killed for food. And that has led us into numbness to the suffering of the animals just to satisfy our lust for meat. How can we be so gentle and loving to our dogs and cats but so unfeeling and blind to the suffering and torture of the animals that grace our plate?

My friend and former pastor, Dr. Adrian Rogers, told this story about a man who had a slaughter house experience similar to mine.

"I heard a man tell a story one time of another man who worked in a slaughterhouse where they butchered cattle. That man thought nothing of his job until one day the slaughterhouse began to process lambs. A lamb came through the chute, and he said, 'It was my responsibility to cut the throat of that lamb.' He said, 'I'd never done that before. I'd watched as the steers would wrestle and fight, but the little lamb just laid his neck back. I put in the knife, and the red blood came out on my hand. The little lamb looked up at me and then licked the blood from my hand.' He said, 'I laid down my knife and resigned my job. I couldn't do it. I could not take the life of a little lamb so meek, so mild.'"[6]

The Lord Jesus came as a lamb and submitted himself for slaughter for us. He did not put up a fight, nor did he utter a word. He is not a martyr. He is the silent Lamb of God who gave Himself for us. Neither the Romans nor the Jews took His life. He gave it willingly.

When we disregard the life that is sacrificed for our hunger for meat, we become less of what God intended for us to be. Let us remember that the animals were given to us for survival and for edification, not for satisfying our lust for flesh. The poorest nations on earth can survive on plant-based diets. Why can't we?

GRACE EXCUSES GLUTTONY?

Christians can be very spiritual on the one hand but very fleshly on the other hand. Our souls are saved by grace, but our bodies are damned by our gluttony and lust. Our souls are saved but our bodies are decimated. Our spirit may identify with Christ but at supper time we give the Lord a tip and dig in with voracity. Just as Gnosticism and Epicureanism are dualisms, Christians are suffering from a split personality. We are stronger at denying the body of extra-marital sex than denying the body of every delectable morsel we see. We have a "see food" diet, and we are hopelessly doomed to physical weakness and early death.

The Apostle Paul hit on this very issue when chastising the disciples about their behavior at the Lord's Supper. The early Christians were letting gluttony and drunkenness destroy the significance of the ordinance of the Lord's Supper.

> Now in this that I declare *unto you* I praise *you* not, that ye come together not for the better, but for the worse. For first of all, when ye come together in the church, I hear that there be divisions among you; and I partly believe it. For there must be also heresies among you, that they which are approved may be made manifest among you. When ye come together therefore into one place, *this* is not to eat the Lord's supper. For in eating every one taketh before *other* his own supper: and one is hungry, and another is drunken. What? have ye not houses to eat and to drink in? or despise ye the church of God, and shame them that have not? What shall I say to you? shall I praise you in this? I praise *you* not.[7]

Too often our ministers try to avoid the possible schism that might result when he brings up a heresy that is becoming widespread. I believe that we, especially Southern Baptists, have avoided a confrontation of the heresy of the New Epicureanism. We have let stand a lust for flesh that is unchristian.

The editor of Creation magazine, David Catchpoole, wrote in an editorial for the June-August issue of 2004 that speaking out as Christians requires courage and steadfastness. **The usual practice today seems to be to avoid confrontation at any cost.** He quotes a bishop's comment on the controversy over his denomination's first homosexual bishop.

"If you must make a choice between heresy and schism", said the bishop, "always choose heresy."[8]

Compromise is very popular today. It is the politically correct action to take in every conflict it seems. But not so in Biblical truth. We must continue to defend the truth of scripture at all costs. Answers In Genesis, the foundation that publishes Creation magazine (Now titled Answers magazine), is determined to defend Genesis from those that would water down the Bible and make it meaningless. **Dr. Catchpoole continues to say that, "By contrast, the bishop's stance (better to choose heresy rather than split the church) was for unity at the expense of truth. That can never be an option for a follower of Christ."**[9]

I pray that our church and denominational leaders will wake up to the physically deadly heresy that has pervaded our Christian faith. A heresy that destroys our "peculiar" denotation as a sanctified body of believers. A heresy that weakens our physical bodies, our witness, and our length of service to our Lord.

---

[1] Tan, Paul Lee. Encyclopedia of 7700 Illustrations : [A Treasury of Illustrations, Anecdotes, Facts and Quotations for Pastors, Teachers and Christian Workers]. Garland TX: Bible Communications, 1996, c1979.

[2] The Holy Bible : King James Version., 1 Ti 4:3. Oak Harbor, WA: Logos Research Systems, Inc., 1995.

[3] The Holy Bible : King James Version., Is 11:6-9. Oak Harbor, WA: Logos Research Systems, Inc., 1995.

[4] The Holy Bible : King James Version., I Cor. 7:1-2. Oak Harbor, WA: Logos Research Systems, Inc., 1995.

[5] This is My Father's World, Maltbie Babcock. Logos Hymnal. 1st edition. Oak Harbor, WA: Logos Research Systems, Inc., 1995.

[6] Proclamation Ornaments Devotional. Rogers, Adrian. Love Worth Finding Ministries. Memphis, TN. 2004.

[7] The Holy Bible : King James Version., 1 Co 11:17-22. Oak Harbor, WA: Logos Research Systems, Inc., 1995.

[8] Duin, J., Heresy better idea than schism? The Washington Times, <washingtontimes.com/national/20040131-12-323-2290r.htm>, 11 March 2004.

[9] Catchpoole, David. Facing the Issue. Creation. Vol. 26, No. 3. p.6.

CHAPTER 9

A FRESH INTERPRETATION

MISINTERPRETATIONS

The following viewpoints are mine. You are free to agree or not to agree with them. However, I believe that they will hold up under scrutiny by theologians who believe in the inerrancy of the cannon of scripture. It appears to me that several key passages in the Bible have been misinterpreted by Baptists, other Christians, and Jews, more by tradition than by true study. This has led us into dangerous lifestyles that lead to early death and dementia. Let us take them one at a time. Some will criticize me for bringing into question the traditional interpretation of these passages. **But it is the traditional interpretations, or misinterpretations that have led us to a blind obedience to a false law of license.** By license, I mean the Merriam-Webster's dictionary definition which says "freedom that allows or is used with irresponsibility", resulting in sickly saints, weak witnesses, obese orators, paltry pastors, miserable missionaries, and all who spend ineffective lives in doctors offices, hospitals, and rest homes, ending in an early arrival at the grave. It is time that we reread these scriptures with an eye to the perfect plan of the Lord Jesus - that of abundant spiritual, intellectual, and physical life here on earth.

Genesis 1:29-30

This is the original diet from the Garden of Eden. God created the world, including the plants and animals that make it a living kingdom. Why did He create the plants first? Scientists tell us that the plants are the only creation that can use photosynthesis to provide food for the animals. No animal can survive without plants. Even so-called carnivorous animals must eat herbivorous (plant–eaters) animals in order to get the nutrition necessary for life. When God finished creation He called it "very good". That means it was perfect. It doesn't get any better than God's "very good". So we can conclude that the original diet was the perfect diet, even for animals such as the tiger, lion, and bear. **Why would God have indicated that in the "peaceable kingdom" there would be no eating of animals by animals if it were not the intended perfect Will of God?** So why can't we go back to that perfect diet today? Well, we are not living in the Garden of Eden, but we can certainly get closer by eating only natural plant foods that God intended for us to eat. **As for me, I want to get as close to God's perfect Will as I can. I do not want to settle for His permissive Will.**

Genesis 9:1-3

In this passage, God gave permission for Noah and his descendants to kill and eat the clean animals for food when the flood was subsided. This was clearly a change in diet for mankind from the original diet of Genesis 1:29-30. In the past few decades we have seen an extraordinary increase in the number of creation scientists. A creation scientist is one who believes in the literal accuracy of the creation account in Genesis of the Bible. If we take their best models, we see that after the flood there was very little live vegetation, except on the ark. All animal life except that in the oceans died and all vegetation was drowned, except for sea plants. Creation scientists also believe that there was an almost global ice age for years after the flood waters receded. Therefore, Noah and his family had very little left to eat when they stepped off the ark. Why then would God save them from drowning to let them die of starvation? In Leviticus 11 God reiterated and expanded upon the rules for eating only clean animals. God allowed them to kill the clean animals for survival and not for health. The animals were given a fear of mankind and mankind was given the freedom to use them for his needs. The age of man dropped to no more than 120 years after this new "Magna Carta" of the post-deluvian world.

Leviticus 11

This passage specifies which animals were safe to consume and allowed to be sacrificed ceremonially. Again, we see that since God gave mankind animals, he also had to protect them by specifying which ones were the more healthy and usable and ones He would accept as unblemished sacrifices. Rather than going into the specific rules of cleanliness and why each animal was qualified or not to be eaten, suffice it to say that God knew which animals were the most dangerous to health as well as which ones were practical as livestock. For Christians these rules were relaxed after the coming of the Messiah since the temple sacrifices were set up to point to the final sacrifice of our Lord. The sacrificial need for animal offerings was forever voided by the one perfect sacrifice of Christ Jesus. The Jews who have rejected Christ as Savior have kept the rules and expanded upon them as Kosher or Kashrut food. There are also some Christian Jews who have continued the Kosher diet, and as a general rule, are healthier than most other Americans.

Some would argue that the unclean animals are not any more healthful than the clean ones, but such may not have been the case back in Old Testament times. Both orthodox Jews and Christian Jews point to the observance of Kosher as building holiness and disciplined living. The fact remains that any animal products, regardless of the degree of harm, are still harmful to health and cannot compare to healthy plant foods. God gave these rules for survival and for ceremony, not for perfect health. Christians are free to eat the animals, but God gives us warnings about which ones are more or less dangerous. In giving us the animals for ceremony and sacrifice, God put limitations on acceptable behavior of the animals He would allow for sacrificial ordinances. **The Levitical Laws, in my opinion, were not the perfect plan for health that God intended from the beginning. They were for discipline, for sanitation, for survival, and for worship, not for optimal health.**

Luke 5:1-11 & John 21:1-14

These two passages are often raised as examples of our Lord Jesus' approval of and participation in meat eating. First, in Luke 5 the Lord goes fishing with Peter, James, and John and uses a splendid analogy to show these new disciples what their mission is to be. These great fishermen had toiled all night and had caught nothing in the Sea of Galilee. So Jesus tells them to go out into the deep and to cast their nets overboard for a catch of fish. Peter tells the Lord that they have fished hard all night without a nibble, but relents out of respect for the Master. Peter probably thought "There are no fish out here, but just to humor the Lord, I'll do what He says." When the nets swelled to almost bursting Peter realizes that His Master of healing and teaching is also Master of the sea and the fish in it. Peter bows down at Jesus' feet and acknowledges that Jesus is Lord of all. They immediately throw down their nets and follow him.

In my opinion, the Lord used this experience to show that He is Lord of the harvest. The harvest of fish is compared to the harvest of souls. **The Lord is not trying to say "Fish are good for you, so go to the fish house every Friday night and gorge yourselves full of them." He is trying to show that when we fish for men, He will provide the catch.**

The second miracle of the catch is in John 21:1-14. The time is after the resurrection when the disciples, Peter, James and John, Thomas, Nathaniel and two other disciples have returned to their fishing for fish. They must have thought that since Jesus had died that their missionary days were over. Well, the Lord changes their minds in a dramatic way as when He first called them on the Sea of Galilee. He sees them out in the water fishing and calls them from the shore. "Children, have ye any meat?" The commentaries say that this greeting is like a customer asking the boys at the meat market if they have any fresh fish. Peter, embarrassed at catching nothing, simply says "No!" The Lord replies, "Cast the net on the right side of ship, and ye shall find". They do as He says and the net bulges with a catch but does not break. John immediately recognizes that it is the Lord. Peter puts on some clothes and dives into the sea toward shore. As they drag the fish to the shore they see that the Lord has a fire going and says "Bring of the fish which ye have now caught. Come and dine". Jesus gives them bread and fish to eat, and then follows the great commission to Peter. Peter, whom the Lord had called to be the leader of the disciples, now is given his final lesson in leadership when Jesus asks him three times "Lovest thou me more than these?...Lovest thou me?...Lovest thou me?" Three times Peter had denied Jesus. Now, three times Peter assures the Lord that he will be faithful.

The first miraculous draught of fishes was to teach the disciples to fish for men. They immediately left their nets and boats and followed the Lord. The second miraculous draught of fishes was to remind them that their calling was to fish for men even though Jesus would not be with them bodily. They left their nets and boats again, but this time they would not return to them, but would follow Him to the end of their lives. They would feed the flock, the church of Jesus Christ. They would feed the church meat (as in deep truth, not just saving bread) just as the Lord was now feeding them meat.

These two miracles of the draughts of fishes were not given to us to give us license to gorge ourselves on animal products. Eating meat is dangerous and not necessary in our day and time. Dig deeper into the Word of God and see that the Lord is telling us that we need to feed the church deep truths and go out into the deep and rescue the perishing and give them meat for their souls, springing up to eternal life.

No Opposition to Meat Eating

Many have said that since the Lord does not preach against meat eating then it must be OK. It is true that He didn't preach against meat eating, and in fact did eat some meat. It is also true that it is not a sin to eat meat. **But to say that the Lord was a meat eater like Americans are meat eaters is a big stretch.** Americans eat meat every meal and the meat they eat is full of hormones, pesticides, antibiotics, bacteria, taste enhancers, chemicals, and worst of all animal fat and cholesterol, which clog their arteries and result in half of all deaths each year in the U.S. Jesus only ate meat during special ceremonies and celebrations if He followed the practice of other Jews of His day. The meat Jesus ate was what we would call organic today. It did not contain the fat and toxins that today's animal products contain. Even today's range-fed livestock still have cholesterol that is deadly for anyone who eats the flesh. And because livestock growers have fed animal flesh back to animals, meat now has deadly prions which causes incurable CJD or Mad Cow Disease in humans.

The occasions where Jesus ate flesh are also occasions where He wanted to identify with mortal men and to relate to them as physical beings. He could not have done that without partaking of cooked flesh as was the tradition of the culture He came to save. He could not have finished the age-old picture of animal sacrifice as instituted in the Garden of Eden if He had not demonstrated approval for animal sacrifice. He was the final sacrifice, pure and holy, and acceptable unto God. **If He had come condemning the killing of animals He would have had to condemn the commandment of sacrificial offerings for sin that He came to fulfill.**

I Timothy 4:4

> For every creature of God *is* good, and nothing to be refused,
> if it be received with thanksgiving: For it is sanctified by the
> word of God and prayer.[1]

This passage has been used for centuries to defend the use of animals for food. I have read commentaries and have seen the research about the consequences of meat-eating. My conclusions on this matter are not arrived at lightly. I agree that God allows and appears to command us to include animals in our diet. **But again I say that even though God has allowed us to eat animal flesh, the underlying reasons for this liberty was for our preservation, our enjoyment, and for tutelage in sacrifice, not so much for longevity of health and wellness.**

This passage warns against those who would fall away from the faith by prohibiting marriage and meat-eating. I have not fallen away from my faith in the Lord Jesus and Him alone for my salvation. But with the whole of scripture in my mind and heart, I am convinced that God wants His bride, the church, to refrain from the life-shortening foods that bring on premature dementia and debilitation during these latter days when He will rapture His bride, the church, at any moment.

Marriage was instituted by God for our proliferation and our salvation, for as Paul has said, it is difficult to live a life totally without sex with the opposite gender. **The fact remains that in heaven, the eternal destination of Christians, there will be no marriage except to the Lamb, and there will be no meat-eating or killing at all.** This proves to me that being disciplined here on earth in marriage and in meat-eating will be two of the highest acts of holiness one could attain. The two most powerful human urges, after air and water, are food and sex. I am not saying that marriage is a sin. It is just a way to avoid sin and at the same time to experience intimacy with another person in a holy way. Neither am I saying that meat-eating is a sin. It was given to us to enable us to survive in this cursed world and to see the picture of sacrifice that Jesus made with His blood and body. **Now that the sacrifice has once and for all been given, there is no reason for the old ceremony to still remain. And there is no reason to continue to eat dangerous foods just to exercise our freedom to do it.**

Because we are weak in the flesh God gave us these two wonderful freedoms. Marriage is a glorious experience when based on love and service to our mate. It is a great exercise in servanthood. Meat-eating is a wonderful culinary delight and brings fullness and satisfaction. It is an experience that reminds us that in this cursed world the death of one allows the life of another, just as Jesus' death gave us life everlasting through faith in Him. Both marriage and meat-eating are freedoms that will not be in heaven, except the marriage to the Lamb. We will have complete communion with the Lord and will never hunger for meat again.

> But drops of grief can ne'er repay
> The debt of love I owe;
> Here, Lord I give myself away,
> 'Tis all that I can do.[2]

I Corinthians 8:8

> But meat commendeth us not to God: for neither, if we eat, are we the better; neither, if we eat not, are we the worse. But take heed lest by any means this liberty of yours become a stumblingblock to them that are weak.[3]

**This scripture from Paul to the Corinthians is intended to assure
the Christians that there was no power of evil in meat that had been
sacrificed to idols because there is no divinity in idols, nor any
power to pollute the soul of the partakers.** Paul addresses a similar
situation in I Cor. 10:25. There is no power of meat to make us any
better in God's sight, or worse. All God's creatures are good as told to
us in Genesis. Verse nine is usually understood to put down the
abstainers of meat-eating as being weak or unlearned. But such is not
the case. This verse was included by Paul to warn those who knew that
the sacrificed meat was harmless but that they should not use this
freedom to become a stumblingblock to those who still admitted that
there was some divinity in that meat because of its use in idol worship.
Many of the Gentile Christians still held onto inclinations of the power
of idols over the meat of sacrifices. So Paul was saying that the liberty
(eating any meat) by strong Christians could lead the weaker Christians
back into the sin of idol worship.

An example might be this: It is general knowledge that many baseball
players are very superstitious about their bats, gloves, clothes, shoes,
shirts, etc. to the point that they have ridiculous rituals that they
religiously follow. Let's say that one has a ritual of wearing the same
undershirt every time he pitches. There is no power whatsoever in an
undershirt to make the pitcher pitch any better, unless it is
psychological. But in the mind of that pitcher, it is a very powerful
force. So he wears it every time he pitches and won't even wash it,
fearing that washing it may reduce its power to help him win games.
This is somewhat the same situation that the Gentile Christians had
concerning meat sacrificed to idols. Their old habits of idol worship and
eating the leftover meat was embedded into their subconscious and had
a powerful influence on them even though they had become Christians.
Paul here in I Corinthians 8 tries to warn them that the meat has no
power in it just as an undershirt has no power to make the pitcher a
winner. He also warns that if we who don't believe in the "power of the
undershirt" start using our "undershirts over and over without washing
them", it would cause the weaker ones to revert back to their old
superstitions.

So Paul is not saying that abstaining from meat is a weakness. He is
saying we should not flaunt our liberty at the peril of weaker Christians.
Meat is not evil in itself. God made it, so it is good, but not necessarily

good for you. Gravity is good, but not good for you if you are falling off a building. Water is good to drink but not good if you are drowning in it. It's the use of good things that make them good or bad. We have used good animals for our gluttony and are paying a tremendous price in lost lives and ministries. **As Christians, we have turned our liberty into a license for over-indulgence and are leading many into disease and death.** Meat-eating is dangerous and not necessary for health in today's world. We have plenty of more healthy fare to enable us to live long and fruitful lives of service to the Lord Jesus Christ.

Acts 10

This scripture is a dramatic story of the great Apostle Peter and how God sent him a vision to instruct him on carrying the gospel to the Gentiles as well as to God's chosen people, the Jews. Peter was a Jew's Jew in that he had observed the ceremonial laws to a tee, especially the laws about clean and unclean animals set down in Leviticus and Deuteronomy. The Gentile, Cornelius, a Roman Centurion, was a Godly man and well thought of by the Jews in Caesarea. God sent an angel to Cornelius and told him to send his servants to get Peter and bring him to his house to instruct him in the gospel. Cornelius did as the angel told him and sent two of his servants and a soldier to Peter's house in Joppa. The next day as the servants of Cornelius were on their journey, Peter was on his rooftop hungry for his noon meal and in prayer to the Lord. At that moment, Peter saw a vision of heaven and a sheet full of all kinds of animals, clean and unclean, being lowered to him.

> And there came a voice to him, Rise, Peter; kill, and eat. But Peter said, Not so, Lord; for I have never eaten any thing that is common or unclean. And the voice *spake* unto him again the second time, What God hath cleansed, *that* call not thou common. This was done thrice: and the vessel was received up again into heaven.[4]

This voice called to him three times because it was directly opposed to what the law of Moses had taught him all his life. Peter was steadfast in the written law and would not obey until confirmation by the angel in repeated commands. Immediately upon completion of the vision the men from Cornelius arrived at his gate. The spirit of the Lord told Peter that the men had arrived and that he was to receive them and to go with them to their master. When Cornelius saw that Peter had arrived he bowed down to Peter.

> But Peter took him up, saying, Stand up; I myself also am a man. And as he talked with him, he went in, and found many that were come together. And he said unto them, Ye know how that it is an unlawful thing for a man that is a Jew to keep company, or come unto one of another nation; but God hath shewed me that I should not call any man common or unclean.[5]

Most theologians interpret this scripture with a two-fold meaning. On the one hand, the ceremonial law of clean and unclean was done away with and on the other hand, the gospel was opened to all nations, the Gentiles as well as the Jews. Of course God can make anything clean if He wants to. He can purge sin from sinners, part the waters, and raise the dead. But I believe that God was not saying, "OK, you can eat anything you want whether it is good for you or not." I believe that God was saying, "There is nothing unclean in and of itself. I made everything and I made it good." In other words, things and people are not good just because they are white Caucasians and bad because they are red Indians, or because they are lambs and not hogs. As the scripture says, "God looketh on the heart, not on the outward appearance". Paul said it this way.

> But he *is* a Jew, which is one inwardly; and circumcision *is that* of the heart, in the spirit, *and* not in the letter; whose praise *is* not of men, but of God.[6]

It is the use of the animal that makes it good or bad. An animal's flesh can become an idol if it is lusted after, becoming gluttony. Animal flesh was given to us for survival and for demonstration's sake. I believe that there is no requirement for us to eat the animals, unless we have no other nutrition available. The healthiest food has been and always will be God's original plant kingdom which was expressly made to nourish our divinely-created bodies. Most of the animal products we eat today have come at great animal suffering brought on by mega livestock farms and industrialized slaughtering with little or no concern for the humane treatment of animals. This, surely, is displeasing to our Saviour, who was born in a feed trough for animals, who rode an animal into Jerusalem, and will ride upon a white horse in His glorious second coming to earth.

Mark 7:14

> And when he had called all the people *unto him*, he said unto them, Hearken unto me every one *of you*, and understand: There is nothing from without a man, that entering into him can defile him: but the things which come out of him, those are they that defile the man. If any man have ears to hear, let him hear.[7]

Some use this scripture to condemn those who fast from meats, those who do so because of the health issue. Jesus was not talking about diet in this passage so much as about the pride of the Pharisees and their legalistic attitudes. The law of Moses was given for cleanliness, health, and ceremonial remembrance of the cleansing of the Holy Spirit. The Pharisees, however, put so much emphasis on the letter of the law that they missed the purpose of the law, that of health and remembrance.

There is no sin in eating or drinking unless our motives are wrong. God gave us food and drink for our health and for our preservation and enjoyment. God did not give us food and drink to abuse by lusting after certain foods and beverages. Lust and gluttony are OUR sins and not the sins of the OBJECTS of our lusts and gluttony. Lust and gluttony come out of us and defile us.

It is not the pistol that kills but the bullet that comes out of the pistol that kills. The trigger of a gun is harmless when there is no cartridge in the chamber. The cartridge is harmless until it is fired from inside the chamber. But when the chamber is loaded with a bullet and the trigger is pulled there comes out a deadly object with terrible consequences. The harm is not from putting the bullet into the gun, but of exploding the cartridge and expelling the bullet. It is what we do with a liberty that makes it a sin or a satisfaction. When Christians eat meat out of lust for it, we cease to become servants and become selfish, disregarding the life sacrificed that allowed us to enjoy it.

Dr. James Dobson was loaded with lots of filth and garbage when he served on Attorney General Edwin Meese's Commission on Pornography, 1985-86. He had to look at some of the most horrible pornography imaginable to understand the degree of filth that had penetrated our public media. But did the same filth come out of him? No. His heart was sealed by the Holy Spirit and these images were blacked out by the power of God to change the heart. That is why we can eat anything and it will not be counted toward us as sin IF we receive it with thankfulness and discernment.

COMING OUT OF SALIVARY SLAVERY

As a Christian who has eaten meat all my life up until a few years ago, I have realized that I don't need to eat meat anymore and I can be healthier without it. I also am convinced that my effectiveness as a Christian and my length of service as such will be extended because of the choices I make in diet and lifestyle. I came to a similar conclusion just after graduating from college at Mississippi State University. I began to drink and smoke and carouse around leaving my first love, the Lord. My mom caught me coming in drunk one night and began to cry. Now I loved my mom more than anything in the world at that time and it broke my heart to break hers. I had seen how my alcoholic father had abused her and night after night had come home drunken and cursing. The Lord broke me right then and there, and from that night on I never touched another drop of alcohol. **I realized that the alcohol had become an idol to me and that what came out of me as a result of drinking it was evil and destructive. I have come to the same conclusion about meats and dairy products. I can live healthy without them because I believe that they lead me into ill health and shortened service to my Lord and Saviour.**

My dad could have been a great Christian leader had not alcohol chained him into slavery to it. He died in his sleep, broken down physically because of his lust for it and his addiction to it. I loved him very much and miss him today as much as I missed him the day that I heard he had died. But his death is not in vain if I can help others to realize that the things that we take into our bodies can result in terrible consequences when they affect what comes out of us. I am convinced that meats, dairy, and poultry products have resulting consequences on the body that are limiting on our service to the Lord Jesus. The toxins that are loaded into our body when we eat these products are stored in our cells where they bring on disease and death. Organic plant foods have no such toxins and will only bring health to our divinely-designed bodies.

PERSECUTION OF PRO-LIVE PEOPLE

It is not popular to promote the live food diet of Genesis 1:29. Those of us who have promoted a return to the original Genesis 1:29 plan of God for dietary wellness have been labeled by some as heretics. Christian vegans have been accused of being legalistic in teaching a return to disciplined living. We have been ignored many times when we mention the fact that dietary discipline can help the body restore itself to health. To our disappointment, the medical community in general has looked upon our ministry with utter disregard and sometimes downright ridicule. There is a general conspiracy of misinformation and a deliberate cover-up of the facts that prove that the plant-based diet of Genesis 1:29 can enable the body to overcome the diseases of our modern culture. Many Christians have been brainwashed by the juggernaut of pseudo intellectualism that claims that the simple plant-based diet is ineffective in bringing health. But plants are anything but simple. Mankind has only begun to scratch the surface of what tremendously complicated synergism of carbohydrates, vitamins, minerals, fats, proteins, micronutrients, enzymes, and even some elements we don't even suspect are included in these beautiful, perfectly-packaged, divinely- created foods.

I submit that the new heresy is actually liberalism resulting in drunkenness and gluttony. Awash in the flood of advertising of processed foods, including animal products, Christians have "let themselves go" when it comes to physical restraint of appetites. The church is no different from worldly persons when it comes to control of appetites. Christians of all denominations are like all Americans who lead the world in Cardio Vascular Disease (CVD), cancer, diabetes, and other degenerative diseases.

WHO IS OUR INTERPRETER?

Because the book of Genesis has been relegated to a fable instead of the inerrant Word of God, the Creator, we are told that the Genesis diet is a thing of the past and is not relevant in today's world. Instead of letting the Bible interpret itself, we have trusted worldly sources. Sometimes these sources are government agencies. Sometimes Christians trust in the very vocations that are supposed to guard our health and well being, such as medical doctors and food and beverage industries. Sadly, we often are led astray by our religious leaders who would rather not rock the boat than spark a revolution in health that could cost them their position as a minister.

It seems that we have opted for the easy way out. In order to protect our idol, fast food (including meats, dairy, sugary desserts, white flour products, and processed foods), we have decided to just find a pill that will remove the disease brought on by our permissive diets. Just look at the ads on prime time television and you'll find a large percentage of them are drug ads. It is truly amazing that we have allowed dangerous pills to proliferate while we suppress healthy alternatives, such as disciplined living and a plant-based diet. Pick up a magazine and chances are you will find pages and pages of drug ads, prescription and over-the-counter ones. The slick ad page is frequently followed by one or two pages of very small print listing the dangers of taking the medication. These ads claim great success over disease but are dangerously masking symptoms, while whole food supplements must carry a label saying something like, "This product is not intended for the treatment, reversal, prevention or cure of disease". **What a joke! The dangerous products have the full protection of the U.S. Government while the very food that God gave us for health must be gagged and tied to a statement of uselessness.** The drug pill ads also include a statement like "Ask your doctor if blankety blank is right for you" to promote the doctors who prescribe them. Ever wonder who the doctor asks? Right! He asks the drug company that manufactures and tests the product. Of course there is no bias in the tests; after all, they are monitored by our FDA!

Past Due Diet Discipline and Live Lifestyle

I believe that it is time for revival of discipline in the church of our Lord Jesus Christ. Far too long Christians have neglected the health and wellness of our bodies in fear that we would be labeled as legalists. Too long have we been reluctant to commit to a vegan lifestyle because it carried with it association with new age philosophy. With better diet and lifestyle, Christians can be healthier and more vital and useable to the work of the Lord. Instead of eating ourselves sick, we can get on with our calling from God - to be the living sacrifice that He designed us to be. Discipline involves being able to withstand temptation. **Until we understand the sources of temptation, the Church of Jesus Christ will never be able to overcome the temptation.**

My favorite Bible teacher is Dr. Adrian Rogers. In his book "Back to the Basics, Volume 1" he reveals sources of temptations we face as Christians. The three sources of our temptations are the **world**, the **flesh**, and the **devil**. His chapter entitled "How to Turn Temptations Into Triumphs" details the problem we all have with our temptations and how to overcome them. He says that we are made in the image of the triune God and we consist of a soul, a body, and a spirit. The world tempts the soul, the flesh tempts the body, and the devil tempts the spirit.

Dr. Rogers says that "the **world**" is referring to the system of evil that we live in, the cursed world. The world tempts the soul or *psyche*. The soul is the mind, will, and emotions of our existence. It is your self, your ego, the person who lives within your body. "It is possible for Christians to become so much a part of this world that they don't stand out for God." It reminds me of the old Royal Ambassador hymn, "The King's Business", which used to be the theme song of the mission program for boys in Southern Baptist Churches.

> I am a stranger here within a foreign land,
> My home is far away, upon a golden strand.
> Ambassador to be, or realms beyond the sea,
> I'm here on business for my King.
> My home is brighter far than Sharon's rosy plain,
> Eternal life and joy throughout its vast domain.
> My Sovereign bids me tell that mortals there may dwell,

and that's my business for my King.
This is the message that I bring,
A message angels feign would sing.
Oh be ye reconciled, thus saith my God and king,
Oh be ye reconciled to God. [8]

The world primarily tempts the soul with power, wealth, and prestige. The soul is our ego. What we think, feel, and do determine the course of our soul. To overcome the world, it takes **FAITH** in the Lord Jesus Christ. To overcome temptations of conforming to the world, it takes confidence in the Lord and His love for us.

In a dietary sense, I relate this to having faith in God's original foods to bring healing and vitality to life. Remember that God created us to be plant-eaters and our bodies run best on that intricately-designed fuel. Power, wealth, and prestige are no substitute for health. Ask any rich man who is in the hospital suffering from cancer and you'll find that the most important thing in life is his health. Without it he won't have life at all. Our mind, our emotions, and our will can resist the temptations of the world when we fill our hearts with faith in God's word, His will, and His way.

The **flesh** means our disposition to sin. Don't blame sin on the devil. We are the responsible party. Each individual must bear his own burden of sin. Flip Wilson was not the first one to blame sin on the devil when he made popular the remark, "The devil made me do it". The first woman did it when she said, "The serpent beguiled me and I did eat" recorded in Genesis 3:13. If the devil left us to ourselves we would still sin. The flesh tempts our body toward lust, laziness, overindulgence, and sexual immorality. To overcome the flesh we must use **FLIGHT** and flee our youthful lusts for sex or food. When faced with temptations of the flesh, do as Joseph did when Potiphar's wife made a pass at him. He fled, even though he was put in prison and falsely accused. He later was exonerated and put second in command of all Egypt. King David was faced with a similar fleshly temptation when he spotted Bathsheba bathing. Instead of fleeing, he lingered and committed a grave sin of murdering the woman's husband to cover up his adultery.

When you are faced with tempting morsels, flee them and find healthy choices. You will be rewarded with health and wellness rather than imprisonment to disease and dementia. Determine beforehand that you will not linger among the sugary desserts, nor tarry at the roast beef, chicken, or ham. Determine beforehand that you will flee to the live food and feast on its rewards.

The **devil** wars against our spirit, trying to cut us off from our relationship with our Lord and Savior. Our spirit is our sense of God-consciousness just as our soul is our self-consciousness. Pastor Rogers says:

> "You know God through your spirit. Animals have a body and a soul, but no spirit; that's what makes man more than an animal. Man can know God. Man has an innate sense of morality. Man can worship God in spirit and in truth." [9]

To overcome the devil we must **FIGHT** him with the sword of the Spirit, the Word of God. Satan wars against our spirit. Jesus used scripture to fight with Satan in the wilderness temptations. James says if we resist the devil he will flee from us. As pastor Rogers says:

> "You can just say, 'Satan, I bring the blood against you. I resist in the name of the Almighty God. My body is the temple of the Holy Spirit, and you're trespassing on His property. Be gone.' Resist the devil and he will flee from you. Satan doesn't want you to understand the power that you have to overcome temptation, but God does. Be strong in the Lord and in the power of His might." [10]

Use what you have learned about dietary truth to war against the lies that are all around us through pseudo scientists and humanist teachers. Fight the temptations of gluttony with the knowledge of healthy diet and lifestyle. Fasting, prayer, and meditation on God's word will help when you are faced with temptations from the devil.

I believe that we must face the fact that Christians have put too much attention on saving our spirit and our soul and too little attention on saving our body. How do we overcome fleshly temptations? By fleeing them. We must fast from the dangerous foods that lead us into sickness

and death. Pastors must begin to wake their congregations up to the
state of the church in physical health. They must be bold and not timid
in preaching that our Christian duty is to live a life of dietary restraint
instead of one of gluttony and drunkenness. What a refreshing wind
would blow if our leaders were more fit and full of vitality. More of our
time would be spent on reaching the lost, teaching the full gospel of
surrender of soul, spirit, AND body to the Lordship of Christ. We
would have a Saviour AND a Lord whom we lived for sacrificially. Our
praise to the Lord would be continually in our mouths and Christians
would become true living sacrifices.

My Jesus, I love Thee, I know Thou art mine;
For Thee all the follies of sin I resign;
My gracious Redeemer, My Savior art Thou;
If ever I loved Thee, My Jesus 'tis now. [11]

---

[1] *The Holy Bible : King James Version.*, 1 Ti 4:4-5. Oak Harbor, WA: Logos Research Systems, Inc., 1995.

[2] *At the* Cross, Isaac Watts. Logos *Hymnal.* 1st edition. Oak Harbor, WA: Logos Research Systems, Inc., 1995.

[3] *The Holy Bible : King James Version.*, 1 Co 8:8-9. Oak Harbor, WA: Logos Research Systems, Inc., 1995.

[4] *The Holy Bible : King James Version.*, Ac 10:13-16. Oak Harbor, WA: Logos Research Systems, Inc., 1995.

[5] *The Holy Bible : King James Version.*, Ac 10:26-28. Oak Harbor, WA: Logos Research Systems, Inc., 1995.

[6] *The Holy Bible : King James Version.*, Ro 2:29. Oak Harbor, WA: Logos Research Systems, Inc., 1995.

[7] *The Holy Bible : King James Version.*, Mk 7:14-16. Oak Harbor, WA: Logos Research Systems, Inc., 1995.

[8] *The King's Business.* E. Taler Cassel. Flora H. Cassel.

[9] Back to the Basics, Vol. One. Rogers, Dr. Adrian. Walk Through the Bible Ministries. Atlanta, GA.1995.

[10] Back to the Basics, Volume I, Dr. Adrian Rogers. Walk Through the Bible Ministries, Atlanta, Georgia. 1995.

[11] *My Jesus I Love Thee*, William Featherston. Logos Hymnal. 1st Edition. Oak Harbor, WA: Logos Research Systems, Inc., 1995.

CHAPTER 10

T O T A L   P R A I S E

CALLED TO PRAISE

The Ten Commandments became the guide for Godly living after the Exodus. These laws were given to perpetuate and preserve the people of God and to set apart the twelve tribes of Israel for service to Jehovah. Listed and expanded upon in The Pentateuch or Torah, these laws and code of conduct consisted of the first five books of the Old Testament and were the basis of conduct for the Jews up until the time of Messiah. Yahweh chose Israel above all others.

> For what nation *is there so* great, who *hath* God *so* nigh unto them, as the LORD our God *is* in all *things that* we call upon him *for* And what nation *is there so* great, that hath statutes and judgments *so* righteous as all this law, which I set before you this day? [1]

Moses realized how God had singled out the Jewish nation to be God's own chosen. He understood that above all the peoples of the world God had revealed the perfect law to them alone. The law of God is perfect and is truly unattainable. It is a high calling and an honor that we have not earned. But in all the law there is no commandment to praise the Lord other than through our commandment to love Him. Thus, we should continually lift up His name and lovingly praise him as Charles Spurgeon says:

You are bound by the bonds of his love to bless his name so long as you live, and his praise should continually be in your mouth, for you are blessed, in order that you may bless him; "this people have I formed for myself, they shall show forth my praise"; and if you do not praise God, you are not bringing forth the fruit which he, as the Divine Husbandman, has a right to expect at your hands. Let not your harp then hang upon the willows, but take it down, and strive, with a grateful heart, to bring forth its loudest music. Arise and chant his praise. With every morning's dawn, lift up your notes of thanksgiving, and let every setting sun be followed with your song. Girdle the earth with your praises; surround it with an atmosphere of melody, and God himself will hearken from heaven and accept your music. [2]

PRAISE FROM LIPS, LIVES, AND LIMBS

Our praise should not be limited to praise from our lips (what we say), but also praise from our lives (what we are) and limbs (what we do). What we say has a great effect on the world. Christians **affect** our world by our faith in the Lord Jesus. What we **say** holds eternal significance.

But I say unto you, That every idle word that men shall speak, they shall give account thereof in the day of judgment. For by thy words thou shalt be justified, and by thy words thou shalt be condemned. [3]

With our **lips** let us therefore tell others about the miraculous self-healing body we have. God designed us with an immune system that can protect us from disease when fueled with the Designer's perfect fuel – fruits, vegetables, nuts, and seeds. Let us sacrifice our comfort zone for the welfare of others. Christians must tell the diseased brother or sister in Christ that there is a better way to health and wellness than pills, surgery, radiation, and chemo. In a loving manner, we must tell them the good news that, "You don't have to be sick!"[SM]

Let us praise the Lord with our **lives**. Making healthy choices in front of others is very powerful and demonstrates the disciplined living that exemplifies the Christ-filled life. It is no sacrificial witness to overindulge at mealtime. It is not exemplary of the Lord's meekness when Christians become fat and out of shape as a result of unbridled gluttony and lack of exercise. Meekness is bridled strength. Dietary discipline is a much better example of the Lord Jesus than unbridled eating and drinking. Sacrificing our fleshly lusts brings about a holiness that is revealing of our close walk with the Saviour.

Let us praise the Lord with our **limbs**. Doing the right thing at the right time can save a life. Our feet and hands are great tools for the furtherance of the Gospel. Christians can have strong and beautiful legs, feet, arms, and hands when we exercise daily. Weight-bearing exercises can bring us stronger bones and more muscle tone. Jogging and swimming can result in maximum lung capacity and endurance. Rebounding can give our lymph system the needed movement it must have since there is no pump to force the lymph fluid through its courses. The hymn says it well.

> Take my life and let it be
> Consecrated, Lord to Thee;
> Take my moments and my days,
> Let them flow in ceaseless praise.
> Let them flow in ceaseless praise.
>
> Take my hands and let them move
> At the impulse of Thy love.
> Take my feet, and let them be
> Swift and beautiful for Thee;
> Swift and beautiful for Thee.
>
> Take my voice and let me sing
> Always, only, for my King.
> Take my lips and let them be
> Filled with messages from Thee,
> Filled with messages from Thee. [4]

If we are to be living sacrifices, then we must be holy, for nothing could be sacrificed that wasn't holy. Being holy is not easy. It takes a love of the Lord Jesus so strong that we would be embarrassed to fail Him. It requires a reverence that goes beyond fear and reaches unto highest honor and glorious praise.

God chose the Jews to be His instrument of praise, and so we too as Christians should be instruments played out for the glory of the Lord Jesus Christ. We are vessels of His marvelous eternally satisfying water, wherein we thirst no more. We should be the lamp that never goes dark in the stormy night and a sunbeam that shines through the clouds of doubt. The simple song by Sunday school teacher, Nellie Talbot, written circa 1900, says it best.

> "Jesus wants me for a Sunbeam, to shine for Him each day.
> In ev'ry way try to please Him at home, at school, at play.
> A sunbeam, a sunbeam, Jesus wants me for a sunbeam.
> A sunbeam, a sunbeam, I'll be a sunbeam for Him."

It's not complicated at all. It is simple. Shine for Him. The only light we have is His light. So let it shine forth brightly into this dark world. But it is not easy. Oftimes, the simple things in life are the most difficult. It is the same with our bodily habits of eating and drinking. That is why the Lord gave His people, Israel, more explicit directions in the area of eating and drinking.

---

[1] *The Holy Bible : King James Version.*, Dt 4:6-8. Oak Harbor, WA: Logos Research Systems, Inc., 1995.

[2] Spurgeon, C. H. *Morning and Evening : Daily Readings*, September 30 AM. Oak Harbor, WA: Logos Research Systems, Inc., 1995.

[3] *The Holy Bible : King James Version.*, Mt 12:36-37. Oak Harbor, WA: Logos Research Systems, Inc., 1995.

[4] *Take My Life and Let It Be*, Frances Havergal. Logos *Hymnal*. 1st edition. Oak Harbor, WA: Logos Research Systems, Inc., 1995.

CHAPTER 11

SANITATION AND SANCTIFICATION

SANCTIFYING THE SAINTS

As an addition to the Ten Commandments, God gave the Israelites dietary laws that were for their preservation and for their sanctification. These laws stemmed from the earlier designation that God gave to Noah as he gathered the animals into the ark. There were only one set of unclean animals that entered the ark whereas there were seven pairs of clean animals (Theologians are split on whether the scripture meant 7 clean animals or 7 pairs of clean animals in Genesis 7:2). When Noah made the first sacrifice after the ark landed he used clean animals. Then when God set up the sacrificial ceremonial laws for the Tabernacle He specified which animals were to be sacrificed and which ones were not to be used. Later in Leviticus 11 and Deuteronomy 14 God was more explicit in which animals were clean and which were considered unclean.

The purpose of the dietary laws appears to be for sanitation and for sanctification. **Because of the different eating habits and digestive systems of these animals, each kind of animal had a slightly different level of safety for health and respectability as sacrificial animals. Is it a coincidence that the clean animals were peaceful, herbivorous animals and the unclean animals were violent scavengers, omnivorous, and carnivorous? Of course not.**

CLEAN OR UNCLEAN

Clean animals were classified as clean if they completely split the hoof and re-ate predigested food. Some argue that the Bible is wrong and that the camel has split hoofs, but upon further examination the hoof is actually joined so closely as to be considered not divided. Similar argument is made for the hare, whose eating habits are not as well known. The hare does re-eat predigested food by a process called refection, not regurgitation as ruminants (cows, sheep, goats) do. The hare has a special type of dropping that is re-eaten and is re-digested just as ruminants. So the Bible is still correct in saying the rabbits and camels do not fit in with the clean requirements. [1] We do not know why these animals were not permitted to be eaten but trust that God knew something that we are not yet privileged to know. The aquatic animals that were clean were the ones with scales and fins. The others, such as crustaceans or shellfish, which generally are scavengers, and ocean predators, were considered unclean.

When the Israelites came into the Promised Land, they encountered heathen peoples who sacrificed animals and humans to their gods. God's dietary laws and the laws of the sacrifice were given to set the Israelites apart from these ungodly cultures. Since drinking blood and offering swine to the gods was common for the heathen, God expressly forbid these practices.

I also believe that God wanted to use the clean animals as an example of the peaceful, nonviolent lives for which the people of God should be known. So what better example of a peaceful, non-violent, submissive sacrifice is there than a young lamb? Other such parallels can be drawn in sacrificing doves, pigeons, and calves. As for bulls and rams, there is great significance here because of the strength of these animals, which are powerful, yet do not eat other animals. **Strong animals, with perfect bodies, make the best sacrifices, living or dead.** A sickly sacrifice is detestable to the Lord as well as unacceptable. The more valuable the sacrifice, the more highly acceptable the offering. The stronger and purer sacrifice of a Christian, given with praise and thanksgiving, is more acceptable to the Lord Jesus than a weak and tainted one that is given reluctantly and hesitatingly.

HEATHEN INFLUENCES

As the Israelites settled Canaan, God gave them victory after victory because they obeyed Him and gave Him glory. They followed the sacrificial ceremonial laws and the dietary laws. They set themselves apart for the heathen nations and drove them out. With the leadership of Moses and Joshua, the Jews occupied the land that God gave to Abraham and they became free of slavery and domination. But as with all mankind, sooner or later we fall away from God's word and we go our own way. **The pure word and way of God have riches both on earth and in heaven. On the other hand, detours into lust and gluttony always have rewards of slavery and death.**

TEMPLE NEGLECTED

Just as the Tabernacle and Temple were neglected in Old Testament times, so have been the temples of the Lord Jesus Christ in our day. **Our bodies are supposed to house the very Spirit of God Almighty, yet Christians let into our temples the most vile and vain sights, sounds, foods, and beverages.** Television, movies, the internet, video games, radio, digital recordings, junk foods, drugs (illegal, prescription, and over-the-counter), canned and bottled beverages, and even personal care products have polluted, profaned, and pulled down our body temples. God did not continue to dwell in a temple where He is not given first place. He is worthy of the best of rooms, a home set aside for Godly fellowship and ministry. His promise to "never leave you nor forsake you" is conditional. That condition is that we acknowledge the Lord publicly as our Lord. That is why Jesus told the crowd in the Sermon on the Mount that obedience and praise is the prerequisites to the abiding presence of God.

> "Not every one that saith unto me, Lord, Lord, shall enter into the kingdom of heaven; but he that doeth the will of my Father which is in heaven." [2]

[1] Sarfati, Jonathan. *Do Rabbits Chew Their Cud?* Creation **20**(4):56 September 1998. *http://www.answersingenesis.org/creation/v20/i4/rabbits.asp* (August 25, 2005).

[2] *The Holy Bible : King James Version.*, Mt 7:21. Oak Harbor, WA: Logos Research Systems, Inc., 1995.

CHAPTER 12

PROVISIONAL PROMISES

SANCTIFICATION OR SACRILEGE

When Solomon finished the temple and God appeared to him, there came a promise with a provision. God would inhabit his people Israel and his glory would be upon the temple that Solomon had built provided Solomon would continue in obedience and praise of the Lord. But if Solomon did not keep the commandments and honor the Lord, the temple would become a place that demonstrated God's abandonment.

> But if ye turn away, and forsake my statutes and my commandments, which I have set before you, and shall go and serve other gods, and worship them; Then will I pluck them up by the roots out of my land which I have given them; and this house, which I have sanctified for my name, will I cast out of my sight, and will make it *to be* a proverb and a byword among all nations. And this house, which is high, shall be an astonishment to every one that passeth by it; so that he shall say, Why hath the LORD done thus unto this land, and unto this house And it shall be answered, Because they forsook the LORD God of their fathers, which brought them forth out of the land of Egypt, and laid hold on other gods, and worshipped them, and served them: therefore hath he brought all this evil upon them. [1]

We, who have invited Him into our hearts to dwell forever, are God's temple. **If we have accepted Jesus as our Lord as well as our Savior, then we will give Him our body as a living sacrifice and will keep this body in good repair.** We will guard our hearts and our minds and our bodies from evil influences that can become idols. We must guard our souls against other gods who will come into our temples and rob the praise that belongs to God alone. Fasting from dangerous foods and feasting on the best of God's provisions will keep our temples strong. Exercise and fresh, clean air will provide our temples with the nutrition that will keep us strong and disease free. We will be careful to only use safe, organic products for personal hygiene and improvement.

Solomon forsook the statutes and commandments of the Lord and God abandoned the temple. What a sobering thought! Would God abandon our bodies to disease and dementia? I believe in a real sense, He will do just that. Although He will not give our souls up to Satan, He will allow our bodies to become diseased because Christians have disregarded His original diet of health and wellness. A physically sick, weak, and diseased Christian can hardly have the impact of a physically healthy, strong and vital witness for the Lord Jesus.

Of course there are exceptions to this rule. Who can forget the saint who through ignorance has let his or her body be racked with disease from an unhealthy lifestyle? Even though the body has been disabled, the saint keeps on praising the Lord. As a minister I have stood by the bedside of many an ailing Christian who through their illnesses have reflected the Lord Jesus in ways that healthy people cannot do. What greater witness is there than to praise the Lord in the fire, even when the lions of disease roar and tear at the body? Still, in most cases this suffering did not have to be. These ordeals of battle did not have to happen. **Mostly through lack of understanding and knowledge of dietary and lifestyle health do most Christians fall into the rut of slavery to the world's foods.**

The way to keep our temples strong and beautiful is to fast from dangerous foods such as animal flesh and dairy products and shy away from processed foods and beverages that are full of synthetic chemicals, sugar, salt, preservatives, and other artificial ingredients. A diet of fresh, organic fruits, vegetables, nuts, and seeds, augmented with fresh concentrated vegetable juice, is the safest, most nutritious diet known to mankind. A lifestyle of daily exercise such as rebounding, walking, jogging, swimming, aerobics, and weight lifting will bring healthier bones and muscles, keener minds, and more active service to the Lord Jesus. Your temple will be beautiful and healthy and your service to the Lord will be more effective and long.

SIEGES AND WORLDLY CORRUPTION

Christians are under siege just as were the people of God in the Old Testament when they strayed away from the protection and power of the Almighty. Just as the Temple of Solomon was eventually destroyed because of evil influences, our bodies can be utterly destroyed by evil influences also. God punished the divided kingdoms with sieges from worldly nations, ending finally in slavery and dispersion. Genesis 6:3 tells us that God decided to shorten the life spans of mankind to 120 years because of corruption. In Genesis 6:6-7 God promised to destroy all flesh because of sin. But for the grace of God upon Noah and his family, we would not be here today.

STRONG AND LONG, NOT DECREPIT AND CURTATE

Scientists tell us today that our genetic code only allows about 90 cell divisions per lifetime, barring accident or lifestyle disease. That amounts to a limit of 120 or so years of life upon this earth. Because of the bottleneck effect of Noah's family of eight we probably lost the genes that enabled our early ancestors to live past 120 years. Because of the small gene pool on the ark, we probably lost the genes that enable long life spans. [2]

Of course, there were other influences on our longevity such as environmental changes in our atmosphere and protection from radiation. But our diet also has an influence on our length of days. Heart disease, cancer, and diabetes bring an early end to our days, which is just fine with Satan, who seeks to devour us before we are able to bring the Kingdom here on earth.

It is not only length of days that count in our service to the Lord. It is also strength of days. The average age of Americans is roughly 77, but most of us can only look forward to immobility, dementia, and bedridden care in our last days. What a great disappointment to Satan would be a Christian who could be strong and active to his expectant life of almost 120 years. Numerous examples exist among the peoples of the world to verify that plant-based diets enable the human body to live to God's limit of 120.

---

[1] *The Holy Bible : King James Version.*, 2 Ch 7:19-22. Oak Harbor, WA: Logos Research Systems, Inc., 1995.

[2] http://www.answersingenesis.org/creation/v20/i4/years.asp

CHAPTER 13

S L A V E R Y   T O
U N G O D L Y
I N F L U E N C E S

WORLDLY DEPENDENCE

When the Israelites abandoned the Lord, He sent worldly nations to take them captive and to disperse them among the four corners of the globe. **The parallel Christians have to the Jews is that we have forsaken the care of our body temples and have been enslaved to worldly lusts that have resulted in broken temples and weakened soldiers of the cross of Christ.** Among the influences that have diluted our effectiveness among the heathen are these.

Today, when Christians seek advice on health, instead of going to the Bible, we go to the secular media, more specifically the medical community for help. We put great trust in **medical doctors**, who are trained in diagnosing illness and prescribing chemicals, surgery, or radiation for alleviating those symptoms. Often, these doctors are Christians just like you and me, but they have been trained to believe that a germ or bug or bad gene has caused our problem. Their training has usually been lacking in nutritional science and preventive care. Most medical schools require no more than one credit hour of nutritional courses in the curriculum. However, today's doctors are well trained in repair of the body in trauma situations. We have probably the best emergency medical care available.

But when it comes to treatment for a disease, we are sorely lacking because of the influence of the **drug industry** on our medical training. Doctors are rewarded handsomely by the big pharmaceutical companies for prescribing their favorite drugs. The side effects of these dangerous chemicals are pages long and sometimes are so small you can hardly read them. In the worst cases, multiple doctors diagnose multiple drugs that work against each other and can lead to worsening of conditions - and even death!

Christians also depend on the **food industry** to only market safe and nutritious food. Little concern is given to the lack of natural nutrition in packaged foods. Little concern is given to the "liveness" and completeness of packaged foods. Food processors are bound by government rules to sanitize their products to the point that it contains no elements that would spoil. The very thing that makes raw, organic food healthful is that it contains live enzymes and phytonutrients that are ultra sensitive to heat, light, air, and radiation. When the food industry packages their product, they must submit it to high heat, such as pasteurization and radiation. When milk is pasteurized, it must be heated to at least 145 degrees F. for 30 minutes in order to kill the enzymes which could make the milk sour.

When we deny the power of our miraculous bodies to heal themselves, Christians are falling into the same trap that ensnared the Israelites. They depended on foreign alliances to help them out of trouble with neighboring nations. They ignored the God who had sanctified them, strengthened them, and saved them from overwhelming numbers of foes. **Christians are ignoring the miraculous power of our God-designed bodies when we go to the medical doctor instead of to the Bible and God's original diet for health.** Secular society has fooled us into thinking that disease is inevitable. We've been told that animal flesh is a necessity for health, but science has proven that the plant-based diet brings health and wellness. The Framington Health Study, the longest running study of diet and heart disease, is still proving that the plant-based diet is the one most likely to lower risk of heart disease. Dr. William Castelli, past director of the study says:

"Vegetarians have the best diet; they have the lowest rates of coronary heart disease of any group in the country."

Popular Opinion

Because of our slavery to secular opinion, we have been hobbled as Christians. Our government began publishing food guidelines in the early 20th century in an effort to help Americans know the elements of a healthy diet. In the last decade, however, the United States Department of Agriculture has promoted a mythical food pyramid that has been contributing to the disease of our nation. Based on propaganda pushed by the dairy and livestock industry, this false dietary health model has contributed to early death at the hands of heart disease, cancer, diabetes, and other degenerative disease. First published in 1992, the U.S.D.A. food pyramid was based on bread, cereal, rice, and pasta. This basis of nutrition leaves us wide open for diabetes, since most of these products are highly processed, leaving only simple carbohydrates. The vegetable and fruit group occupied the second tier of the pyramid, but should be the ground floor of any healthy diet. The big problem with this pyramid is the inclusion of the third tier consisting of dairy and meat products for a total of as much as six servings a day, enough to guarantee that the practice of this diet will lead to CVD and cancer. The evidence is conclusive that this diet has resulted in the statistic that one of every two Americans will die of heart disease. Throughout this pyramid there is the inclusion of added sugar and added fats, which contribute to diabetes and other degenerative diseases.

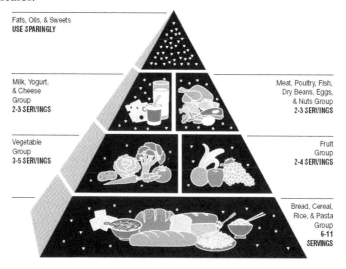

Fats, Oils, & Sweets
USE SPARINGLY

Milk, Yogurt,
& Cheese
Group
2-3 SERVINGS

Meat, Poultry, Fish,
Dry Beans, Eggs,
& Nuts Group
2-3 SERVINGS

Vegetable
Group
3-5 SERVINGS

Fruit
Group
2-4 SERVINGS

Bread, Cereal,
Rice, & Pasta
Group
**6-11
SERVINGS**

Since 1894 the United States Department of Agriculture has sought to
help Americans to know the foods that are necessary for health by
publishing Food Guidelines. Too many times they have disregarded the
original diet from God and have followed the Plan B diet including
meats and dairy and processed and packaged foods. 2004 was a year of
reassessing the dietary needs of Americans by that same USDA.
Hearings have been held and a wide variety of input from all interests
have been compiled and considered. To their credit, they are sensitive
to the state of ill health of our nation. But in the spring of 2005 they
again caved in to the powerful food industry and developed not one
pyramid, but a "take your pick" group of pyramids. By giving people a
choice of which pyramid they desire, the USDA has copped out on their
responsibility to provide scientific guidance to Americans and the world
concerning healthy diet and lifestyle. They have again yielded to the
unscientific propaganda that for years has blinded America and the
world to the dangers of meat, dairy, and processed foods, full of
additives and chemicals. I am afraid that we will continue to lose the
battle for the body, unless more voices are raised that bring us back to
the Garden diet of plant based nutrition.

DETERIORATION TO DESTRUCTION TO RECONSTRUCTION

Christians have become like the kingdom of Judah of the Old
Testament. The southern kingdom had gone through king after king,
some good and some bad. The gradual deterioration of the temple had
resulted in it being desecrated by King Ahaz when he set up a shrine to
the god of Syria inside the temple. Following Ahaz, Hezekiah became
one of the best kings of the southern kingdom of Judah.

For good King Hezekiah, the restoration of the temple after the reign of
Ahaz, the second most terrible king of the Southern Kingdom of Judah,
was an emotional experience. Under Ahaz, who sacrificed his own son
to a heathen god, the kingdom of Judah and the temple were both
brought into disarray and pollution. In II Chronicles we see that King
Hezekiah, in an effort to return Judah and the temple to the worship of
the one true God, brought the people together for a Passover, even
though the time was not right. Those priests and people were not fully
sanctified and purified for service. But God, because of his great love
and forgiveness, allowed the observance of the Passover and a return to
temple worship.

For a multitude of the people, *even* many of Ephraim, and Manasseh, Issachar, and Zebulun, had not cleansed themselves, yet did they eat the passover otherwise than it was written. But Hezekiah prayed for them, saying, The good LORD pardon every one *That* prepareth his heart to seek God, the LORD God of his fathers, though *he be* not *cleansed* according to the purification of the sanctuary. And the LORD hearkened to Hezekiah, and healed the people.? [4]

When the captives returned from Persia with Nehemiah, they immediately rebuilt the foundation of the temple that had been destroyed by the Babylonians. Under Zerubbabel, the governor, the foundation was rebuilt and a great celebration ensued. The old men, who had seen the temple in its splendor, now wept at the sight of the limitations of this second temple. **While the younger people praised the Lord for hope of a new temple, the older ones lifted up cries of sorrow because the new temple would not measure up to the original one due to their sin and corruption.**

But many of the priests and Levites and chief of the fathers, *who were* ancient men, that had seen the first house, when the foundation of this house was laid before their eyes, wept with a loud voice; and many shouted aloud for joy: So that the people could not discern the noise of the shout of joy from the noise of the weeping of the people: for the people shouted with a loud shout, and the noise was heard afar off. [5]

What a parallel this event is to the plight of our body temples today! Christians have neglected God's perfect diet and have imbibed in the world's food idols. Fast, fatty foods have replaced the nutrient-rich and fiber-loaded natural foods which God intended for us to thrive on. Animal products have drastically lowered our quality of physical life and limited our life spans. Our authorities are the medical and drug companies instead of the Lord God Almighty and His Holy Word. **Our temples have deteriorated to the point that they are but a shadow of the lean, muscular frames of our pre-flood ancestors.**

Christians are losing the battle for their body temples. Praise be to God we have the spiritual victory over sin and death through Jesus Christ our Lord - but our earthly ministry is weak because of our physical weakness and shortness of effective service to the Lord due to our diets and lifestyles. We have seen our temples cheapened, weakened, torn down, and destroyed by the worldly food for which we have lusted. The idols of our day are fast food, beverages, money, automobiles, clothes, sports and athletes, houses, television, recreation, movies and movie stars, and pornography. The Christian church has put many things ahead of our love for the Lord Jesus Christ, and we are paying for it by slavery to the world, just as the Northern and Southern Kingdoms of the Old Testament experienced.

His Mercy Is Everlasting, His Truth Endureth to All Generations

But there is hope. Our miraculous, self-healing bodies can and will restore themselves when we fast from the dangerous foods and feast on God's original recipe for health. **The battle can be won. Our weapons are fresh fruits (preferably organic) , raw vegetables (preferably organic), raw nuts and seeds, pure water, organic personal care items, daily exercise, fresh clean air, sunshine, rest, and meditation upon the Word of God. (I also include fresh vegetable juice as a part of my regimen – at least two cups daily.)** With these weapons of wellness, Christians, the bride of Christ, can again restore the house of the Lord, our body temples. We can vow, as did the enslaved remnant returning to the destroyed temple in Jerusalem (Nehemiah 10:39), "and we will not forsake the house of our God".

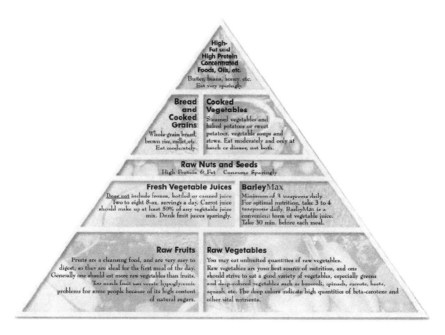

This food pyramid from Hallelujah Acres is very close to the original Garden diet with the addition of the fresh vegetable juices. Thousands are returning to health by following this map for optimal nutrition. Used by permission of Hallelujah Acres, Inc.

---

[1] http://www.idfa.org/facts/milk/pasteur.cfm

[2] The Hallelujah Health Tip(SM)Issue #367: The Maker's Diet; A Critique by Rev. Malkmus(Part 10)November 30, 2004.

[3] http://www.nal.usda.gov/fnic/Fpyr/pyramid.html

[4] *The Holy Bible : King James Version.*, 2 Ch 30:18-20. Oak Harbor, WA: Logos Research Systems, Inc., 1995.

[5] *The Holy Bible : King James Version.*, Ezr 3:12-13. Oak Harbor, WA: Logos Research Systems, Inc., 1995.

CHAPTER 14

R E B I R T H   A N D
R E G E N E R A T I O N

Restoring Rotten Fruit

Today's Christians are rotting on the vine. We must get our bodies back
into health and wellness so that we might be the spotless bride of Christ.
Time is short and the Groom could come at any moment!(Matthew
25:1-13) Let us begin the restoration immediately. The wall must be
rebuilt to keep out the enemy that can destroy us.(Nehemiah 3:1-32)
We have a fantastic body that can literally rebuild itself when given the
right materials. The wall of wellness must be restored and can be
restored by disciplined living and a constant fast from worldly poisons.
Testimonies abound that verify the fact that the plant-based diet can
return the body to health from virtually any degenerative disease.

Planted in Rich Soil

Hallelujah Acres web site (www.hacres.com) is loaded with experiences
of Christians who have returned to the Garden diet, augmented with
fresh vegetable juices and pure water. Thousands and thousands have
lost weight, regained strength, extended their lives, and become more
effective as gospel missionaries. The author's own web site
(www.aofood.com) contains help for those who would determine to fast
from the world's poisons and feast on the Garden menu of whole, live
foods that can enable the body to heal itself.

For more scientific proof of the benefits of the plant-based diet, there are numerous sources that are trustworthy.   The aforementioned Physicians Committee for Responsible Medicine (www.pcrm.org) is a valuable professional organization that is at the forefront of research and publication of plant-based diet data. Founded by Dr. Neal Barnard, this organization is leading the charge of physicians to a return to the ministry of healing by prevention instead of side-effect-laden medications.

Medical doctors who are returning to a ministry of "preventive medicine" are experiencing tremendous results when they incorporate the plant- based diet into their medical practice. Men such as Dr. John McDougall   (www.drmcdougall.com),   Dr.   Joel   Fuhrman (www.drfuhrman.com),   and   Dr.   Caldwell   Esselstyn (www.heartattackproof.com) have demonstrated that the plant-based diet is the only way to health and wellness.

Research by renowned Ph. D.'s, such as Dr. T. Colin Campbell, has also strengthened the cause of the return to natural diets and lifestyles. Dr. Campbell's China Project (www.vegsource.com/event/campbell.htm) has provided the first long term, wide spectrum, documented evidence that the animal diet does detrimentally affect health and longevity. His new book, The China Study, has been hailed by the *New York Times* as "The most comprehensive large study ever undertaken of the relationship between diet and the risk of developing disease". [1]

WATERED WITH THE WORD

Daily study and meditation on the Word of God is vital for a healthy soul, spirit, and body. We are three entities sort of like the Trinity of Father, Son, and Holy Ghost. We have a living soul, a unique spirit, and a beautiful body that must live in concert to accomplish the wonderful symphony that God has composed us to be. Caring for all three of these aspects of our being is a daily task. Let us feed our souls with faith from God's word, our spirits with praise of our Creator, and our bodies with Garden food.

Fertilized with Living Nutrition

Our bodies must have live food - food that is raw, fresh, and full of nutrition. Organically-grown food has a wide spectrum of micro and macro nutrients that God has designed to furnish perfect fuel for us. Cooked food is dead food, void of the enzymes that cannot live above 107 degrees Fahrenheit and weakened by the denatured protein and limp fiber that result from cooking food. **Christians have to break the habit of cooking our foods and relearn the art of preparing foods without destroying the nutrition naturally contained therein.**

Start now in building your library with recipes of raw and lightly-cooked foods. My wife, Marilyn, a trained Health Minister, has just finished writing a book, Hallelujah! Simple Easy Meal Plans, which includes weekly grocery lists and menus for each week of a month, so that even the beginner in healthy nutrition can prepare healthy meals. In my bibliography are some recommended sources of ways to prepare great-tasting, satisfying, and nutritious foods. Begin now to rid your kitchen of the deadly packaged foods and animal products that bring disease and dementia to our body temples. Get a garbage bag and collect them all to either throw away or give to those who don't have any food at all. Then stock your pantry with healthy foods. You might want to buy another refrigerator to keep the fresh fruits, vegetables, nuts and seeds that you will be stocking. Helpful machines like a water distiller, masticating juicer, food processor, dehydrator, and blender will help also. See our web site at http://www.aofood.com for suggestions.

Strengthened by Testing

Trees grow stronger by the testing of the wind and the beating of the rain upon them. The sunshine toughens the bark and provides the catalyst for the wonderful chemical reaction of photosynthesis that enables life. So too does our body grow strong and supple when we test it by exercise, fresh air and sunshine.

Sunshine is the magic ingredient that enables our body to make Vitamin D, the regulator of calcification and decalcification in our structural framework. In The China Study, Dr. T. Colin Campbell reveals that as the latitude increases and the sunshine exposure decreases so does the incidence of multiple sclerosis, MS. It is important to get at least 30 minutes of sunshine each day on your skin to allow this process to work properly.

There are three forms of exercise that provide a balanced approach to strengthening the body. The first is **stretching**. This prepares the muscles, tendons, and joints for the extended movement that is coming. The second is **aerobics** exercise, which challenges the heart to beat faster and the lungs to work more efficiently. Aerobic exercise for one hour should be a part of every day's activities. The third exercise is strength training or **resistance training**. This type of exercise is proven to increase joint strength and muscle mass. Research has proven that resistance training extends life span. It is essential to alternate the work out to different muscle groups each day so that repair and rebuilding are allowed. Lastly, a **cool down** period helps the body to recover.

Remember, that a great diet without exercise is just as bad as a bad diet with great exercise. Strive for both perfect diet and regular exercise in your daily regimen. Establish a regimen by practicing it for 21 days. Research shows that actions become habits when consistently practiced for three weeks. When you have established a habitual regimen it is much easier to keep with the program.

GROW NOW THAT YOU ARE PLANTED

Our growth as Christians is likened unto the growth of a seed into a mature, strong tree, yielding much fruit and proliferating itself through the spreading of the seed. We are the fruit of the work and witness of other Christians. Someone told us the Gospel story and the Holy Spirit of Christ Jesus drew us toward Him. We were convicted of our lost condition, made a public profession of our faith in Jesus and were baptized as a picture of our death to sin and rebirth to eternal life in Christ. Thus began our growth as Christians.

Consider yourself as a seed. As a seed, you died. Only then could you be reborn as a seedling. Cut off from the life-giving plant, your enzyme inhibitors prevented you from having life. Then, you were nurtured with warm, moist, and fertile soil until the enzyme inhibitors in the seed were broken open and you sprouted into a young, tender seedling.

Protected form the extremes of temperature and wind, you grew. As you developed stronger stem and more advanced leaves, you also developed a wider root system of support. You required more nutrition and more water for continued sustenance. Then the day came when you could be tenderly uprooted and placed in the ground outside among the mature trees. No longer were you protected from the wind and extreme weather. You grew stronger because of the testing of your roots and your stems and leaves. Now you had to go deeper into the soil for more support and more water for your growing branches. The sunshine and rain helped you to develop flowers that attracted bees and butterflies that fertilized them as they spread your pollen to nourish other trees and to develop other's fruit. Your fruit was set because you shared your pollen as did the other trees. Soon your flowers developed into tiny fruit that had the promise of ripening. More rain, sunshine, minerals from the ground and the chemical factory God put into your genetic code produced perfect fruit. As the days passed the fruit ripened and turned into glorious colors that trumpeted "pick me, I'm ready to eat". Finally, you were picked and you were eaten so that others might live.

Correspondingly, our lives as Christians have traveled a similar path. We must die to self before we can live to Christ. We start out our Christian lives as tiny seeds inhibited by the world. As other Christians love us and teach us, we are broken and we realize our desperate condition. A sprout of love for Jesus breaks through our hard hearts and we begin to mature as babies. We are slowly fed by friends and fellow Christians with knowledge of our Savior through Bible study and teaching. As our hearts grow stronger and our knowledge of the Lord increases, we grow taller and more solid in our faith and we are more deeply rooted in the soil of Christian doctrine. Soon we are able to stand the temptations of the world and we are fruit bearers. We are picked at the peak of ripeness to feed the hungry and to furnish seed for other generations. Many are led to sprout into Gospel messengers and missionaries because of our one seed that carried the message of salvation. The law of the harvest is fulfilled.

> Be not deceived; God is not mocked: for whatsoever a man soweth, that shall he also reap. For he that soweth to his flesh shall of the flesh reap corruption; but he that soweth to the Spirit shall of the Spirit reap life everlasting. And let us not

be weary in well doing: for in due season we shall reap, if we faint not. As we have therefore opportunity, let us do good unto all *men*, especially unto them who are of the household of faith. [2]

Don Wildmon, founder of the American Family Association, tells the story illustrating this scripture in his booklet <u>Nuggets of Gold.</u> The American Family Association web site is <u>www.afa.net.</u> In the story entitled "Be Careful What you Build" he tells of a rich man who came to his friend, a building contractor, and told him that he was going on an extended vacation and wanted a house to be built for him while he was gone. "Spare no expense in materials and workmanship," the rich man said, "and I will pay you well." So the rich man went on his vacation and the contractor began building the mansion. Now the contractor reasoned within himself that this rich friend would not be able to tell the quality of materials in his new home for he was not knowledgeable in building materials or methods. The contractor would be able to make a lot of money off the rich man and still have a beautiful home although time would eventually tell that inferior materials had been used in its construction. The rich man finished his vacation, called the contractor, and arranged to see the completed mansion. Arriving at the new home, the contractor assured the rich man that he had spared no expense in building the house, but that it had cost much more than he had anticipated. The rich man said that he understood and that he had expected to pay more. As they finished the inspection the rich man turned to his friend, the contractor, and said, "John, we have been friends for a long time. I have looked for some way to express my love for you and your family. I'm getting on in years and I wanted to do something for you before I die. Here is the deed to the land and the keys to the house you have built. You built it, now you can live in it."

Our body is our house where we invite Jesus Christ, our Lord, to live. If we skimp on fuel for our body house, our temple for the Holy Spirit, we cheapen it and it will deteriorate rapidly. When we build a cheap house we will live in a broken down temple. **Let's build a mansion for our Lord, a temple that is well kept and built strong as a result of consuming the very best foods we can find. Sow healthy foods and active lifestyle and you will reap a strong, healthy body, soul, and spirit.**

RIPEN THAT YOU MAY BE PICKED

In a similar way, let me encourage you to grow and mature in your knowledge of health and nutrition. You have seen the light of truth in this book. You have sprouted and taken root in the knowledge of how to be healthy and well. Hopefully, you will continue to be fed and nurtured with the truth of God's original diet for health and healing. Please pray for more wisdom to know the truth and you will be set free indeed. **There is a wonderful feeling of freedom when you realize that you have the power to be free of cancer, heart disease, diabetes, and all other degenerative diseases by simply changing what you eat and drink.**

But just as the seedling must be buffeted and tested, you will be buffeted and tested. There will be healing crises that will come when your body begins the detoxification process of ridding itself of the toxins that have built up over years of eating animal products and processed foods. There will be detractors who will preach to you that the Bible commands us to eat meat. Don't believe them. God allows us to eat meat just as He allows us to jump off a cliff, or to divorce our spouse, or to have servants, or to marry whomever we choose, etc. But there are decisions that are downright unwise and will lead to consequences of ill health and broken lives. One of those decisions is the choice of animal flesh as food. We don't need it! We don't have to have it for health! We can have much better health without it. Animal sacrifice is no longer needed for our survival, or our edification. If we are found without fresh produce, we can eat meat as a survival option. Remember, God gave us the animals for our benefit, not for our exploitation.

Oswald Chambers gives us guidance in his book, <u>My Utmost for His Highest,</u> on how to win the battle for the body in the daily devotion for December 27. **The battle plan must be decided upon in the heart before the battle can be won in the world.**

Where the battle's lost and won
If thou wilt return, O Israel, saith the Lord
Jeremiah 4:1.

The battle is lost or won in the secret places of the will before God, never first in the external world. The Spirit of God apprehends me and I am obliged to get alone with God and fight the battle out before Him. Until this is done, I lose every time. The battle may take one minute or a year, that will depend on me, not on God; but it must be wrestled out alone before God, and I must resolutely go through the hell of a renunciation before Him. Nothing has any power over the man who has fought out the battle before God and won there. If I say—'I will wait till I get into the circumstances and then put God to the test,' I shall find I cannot. I must get the thing settled between myself and God in the secret places of my soul where no stranger intermeddles, and then I can go forth with the certainty that the battle is won. Lose it there, and calamity and disaster and upset are as sure as God's decree. The reason the battle is not won is because I try to win it in the external world first. Get alone with God, fight it out before Him, settle the matter there once and for all.[3]

Temptations can be overcome if anticipated and settled before the battle begins. **Decide which foods you will eat and which foods you will not eat. Rehearse the reasons for eliminating that food and get God's advice before you face the test. The Lord deserves our best commitment, our living sacrifice, our utmost for His highest glory.**

There will be temptations to eat highly-processed foods that contain dangerous chemicals, preservatives, and food additives. In his book, Excitotoxins, The Taste That Kills, noted brain surgeon, Dr. Russell Blalock warns against MSG and similar taste enhancers that are contained in most salad dressings and a host of other foods, including soups. His warnings include a conviction that these additives are a major cause of brain damage and lead to dementia such as Alzheimer's disease, Lou Gehrig's disease, and Parkinson's disease.[4]

There will also be detractors to the original diet that will say things like, "It's too restrictive", or "I just can't live like that", or "I've got to have my meat". Realize that this sort of thinking is rebellious to the plan of

God; that we be a living sacrifice, not an unbridled runaway. Some will say that the plant-based diet is incomplete without meat and dairy. The meat and dairy industries conduct short term research that they hope will prove that meat and dairy products are necessary for health. They do not want the public to believe that the plant-based diet is sufficient for healthy living. They do not want you to know about independent long-range studies over years and years of research and even thousands of short term studies that prove that the plant-based diet is the only way to health and wellness.

Another unwise decision is the neglect of exercise and fresh air. Without exercise and fresh air, the body will wither and become diseased. When the space program was just getting underway, our astronauts learned the importance of exercise. In 14 days in space the men lost almost 15% of their muscle and bone mass. Exercise is vital for developing bone density and muscle mass. Walking is great exercise and almost anyone can do it indoors (with a treadmill or at a mall) or outdoors on a track or neighborhood trail. Another suggestion is a rebounder, a small trampoline that offers great exercise at any level of physical ability. Whether it be home exercise or membership in a health club, it is wise to schedule daily exercise and make it a habit. Exercise should include a warm up period (stretching), aerobics (elevation of heart rate and respiration), resistance exercise (weights), and a cool down period. The apostle Paul knew the necessity of training.

> Know ye not that they which run in a race run all, but one receiveth the prize? So run, that ye may obtain. And every man that striveth for the mastery is temperate in all things. Now they *do it* to obtain a corruptible crown; but we an incorruptible. I therefore so run, not as uncertainly; so fight I, not as one that beateth the air: But I keep under my body, and bring *it* into subjection: lest that by any means, when I have preached to others, I myself should be a castaway. [5]

Remember that a large percentage of our nutrition comes from the air we breathe. Therefore, it is vital to get fresh air along with your daily exercise. Polluted air is not just outside air. The EPA has recognized the seriousness of indoor air pollution.

In the last several years, a growing body of scientific evidence has indicated that the air within homes and other buildings can be more seriously polluted than the outdoor air in even the largest and most industrialized cities. Other research indicates that people spend approximately 90 percent of their time indoors. Thus, for many people, the risks to health may be greater due to exposure to air pollution indoors than outdoors. [6]

An indoor air purifier is a good idea. See our web site, www.aofood.com, for more information about indoor air purification products.

Sunshine has been given a bad rap because of the trans fatty acids that we consume in snacks and fast foods. These fats accumulate under the skin and can turn into carcinogens when struck by the rays of the sun. Baylor College of Medicine in Houston has proof of this fact. In May of 2003, Dr. John Wolf, chair of the department of dermatology at Baylor College of Medicine relayed these findings:

> An unexpected way of lowering your risk of skin cancer is to eat a low-fat diet, said Wolf. In 1994, he and other members of his department published the results of a federally sponsored study that evaluated the effect of a low-fat diet on the occurrence of precancerous skin lesions called actinic keratoses.
>
> The researchers randomly assigned 76 patients to eat their usual diet (approximately 40 percent fat) or a diet that was 20 percent fat. During the two-year study, physicians who did not know which diet the patients were following examined the patients for new actinic keratoses.
>
> In months 4 through 24, there was an average of three new actinic keratoses per patient in the group on the low-fat diet and 10 in the group on the high-fat diet. *(New Engl J Med 330:1272-1275 May 5, 1994)* [7]

Such research as this is readily available on the internet, in books, videos and other sources. Become fully developed in the faith of wellness and teach it to others that your faith will be strengthened and the secret of physical health will be spread abroad. This author and his wife regularly teach Biblically based The Hallelujah Diet and Lifestyle®, whose web site is at http://www.hacres.com, We teach a nine week seminar entitled "Get Healthy! Stay Balanced", a weekend retreat titled "Back to Life", and also hope to open a local resource center soon in Jackson, TN. Our web site http://www.aofood.com is a good source of new information on how to return to health God's way.

SPREAD THE SEED OF SALVATION

Now that you have read this book, you have a great responsibility. You have a treasure that must be shared. It is an awesome knowledge that you now have. **Just think. You have the knowledge and the Biblical background to never fear physical illness again!** The degenerative diseases that beset Americans cannot harm you if you stay the course of natural health through God's perfect diet. You now have the secret to living a healthy 120 years and more! Except for accidents or bodily injury, you can have a healthy life, a life more abundant in every way.

You now have a three-pronged gospel, not just a single gospel of spirit regeneration. Your soul, spirit, and body now can be spared the degradation that affects most of our nation and world. With the renewed faith in the Genesis diet, you can avoid the illnesses and weaknesses of the world's diet. Your gospel is that "You don't have to be sick!" Shout it from the mountain tops!

Only Jesus saves! And He saves soul, spirit, AND body! It is a marvelous gospel. It is a freeing message that can bring renewed hope to a hopeless world. The knowledge you now have must be scattered abroad to neighborhoods and nations. Christians arise! To the work, to the work!

THE VISION OF VICTORY

I see a new day coming for the church of the Lord Jesus Christ. The bride of Christ is adorned in health as the world grows sicker. There is a Health Minister in every church who teaches and organizes classes in

Biblical nutrition. Bold yet caring pastors include messages to their congregations on dietary discipline and self control in appetites. I see Christian doctors lead the way in a return to preventive health care through improved diet and lifestyle. My vision sees drugs and medical intervention minimized and taken as a last resort. Church meetings are balanced with fasting as well as feasting and celebration. Fervent, effectual prayer has returned. The church is healthier and there is more opportunity to pray for spiritual needs rather than physical ones. Instead of long lists of sick, there are long lists of needs for spiritual deliverance. Christians now have a reputation for wellness and vitality in spiritual, intellectual, AND physical activities. Lastly, I see the bride of Christ, His glorious church, strong and healthy as the time approaches for the glorious wedding feast of the Lamb of God. This vision can become reality if we will only go back to the original diet from Genesis 1:29.

There's a battle raging throughout all of the world
for the temple of the Lord most high.
Not the temple of the desert or the temple on the hill,
but the one in which we live or die.

There's a battle royal for the bodies of the saved
and it's fought a most unusual way.
Not with rocket launchers, laser bombs, nor supersonic jets
But how we eat, drink, work, rest and pray.

For we battle not against another's flesh and blood,
But our war is private and within.
No, we fight against the gluttony and tastes the world promotes,
And against our body's selfish whim.

Let us win this battle for the glory of God
For Christ's Bride should strong and spotless be.
Not diseased and sickly, tired and lifeless, overweight and fat;
But a strong and healthy house, disease free.

The Battle for the body must be won today,
Because Satan wants us weak and lame.
Let us feast upon the plant foods God designed for us,
Strong and healthy, we will bless His name.[8]

[1] The China Study, T. Colin Campbell, PhD, Benbella Books, Dallas, Texas, 2004.

[2] *The Holy Bible : King James Version.*, Ga 6:7-10. Oak Harbor, WA: Logos Research Systems, Inc., 1995.

[3] Taken from *My Utmost for His Highest* by Oswald Chambers, © 1935 by Dodd Mead & Co., renewed © 1963 by the Oswald Chambers Publications Assn., Ltd. Used by permission of Discovery House Publishers, Box 3566, Grand Rapids MI 49501. All rights reserved.

[4] Excitotoxins: The Taste That Kills, Blalock, Russell, M.D., Health Press, Sante, New Mexico, 1997.

[5] *The Holy Bible : King James Version.*, 1 Co 9:24-27. Oak Harbor, WA: Logos Research Systems, Inc., 1995.

[6] IAQ Publications, *Indoor Air Concerns*, *http://www.epa.gov/iaq/pubs/insidest.html#Intro1* (August 27, 2005).

[7] http://www.bcmfindings.net/vol1/is5/03may_n2.htm

[8] Poem by the Author, Doug Polk *Battle for the Body* by Doug Polk, 2006

BIBLIOGRAPHY

(Please be aware that some of these books are by authors who are not evangelical Christians. Still, they all contain valuable information that enforces the plant based diet and lifestyle of Genesis 1:29)

Appleton, Nancy. *Lick the Sugar Habit*. Santa Monica, CA: Avery, 1996.

Balch, Phyllis A.and James F. Falch. *Prescription for Nutritional Healing,* 3rd ed., New York: Avery, 2000.

Banik, Allen E. *The Choice Is Clear*. Austin, TX: Acres U.S.A., 1989.

Bartholomew, Mel. *Square Foot Gardening*. Emmaus, PA: Rodale Press, 1981.

Bieler, Henry G. *Food Is Your Best Medicine*. New York: Ballantine Books, 1992.

Blaylock, Russell. *Excitotoxins The Taste That Kills*. Sante Fe, NM: Health Press. 1997.

Campbell, T. Colin. *The China Study*. Dallas: BenBella Books, 2005.

Catchpoole, David. Facing the Issue. *Creation*, June-August 2004, p.6.

Chambers, Oswald. *My Utmost for His Highest*. Grand Rapids: Discovery House Publishers, 1963.

Erasmus, Udo. *Fats that Heal, Fats that Kill.*, Burnaby, BC, Canada: Alive Books, 1993.

Foster, Cynthia A. *Stop the Medicine*. Scottsdale, AZ: Break On
Through Press, LLC, 1999.

Fuhrman, Joel. *Eat to Live*. Boston: Little, Brown and Company, 2003.

Fuhrman, Joel. *Fasting and Eating for Health*. New York: St. Martin's
Press, 1995.

Ham, Ken A. *The Lie Evolution*. El Cajon, CA: Creation-Life Publishers, 1987.

Howell, Edward. *Enzyme Nutrition, The Food Enzyme Concept*.
Wayne, NJ: Avery Publishing Group, Inc.1985.

Hudson, Robert. *The Christian Writer's Manual of Style*. Grand Rapids:
Zondervan, 2004.

Hulse, Virgil. *Mad Cows and Milk Gate*. Phoenix, OR:
Marble Mountain Publishing, 1996.

Idol, Olin. *Pregnancy, Children, and The Hallelujah Diet*.
Shelby, N.C.: Hallelujah Acres, 2002.

Jeavons, John. *How to Grow More Vegetables*. Berkeley, CA: Ten Speed
Press, 1995.

Lee, John R. *What Your Doctor May Not Tell You About
Menopause*. New York: Warner Books, Inc., 1996.

Lyman, Howard F. *Mad Cowboy*. New York: Simon & Schuster, Inc., 1998.

Lyman, Howard. *The Truth About Meat and Dairy*. VHS Video. Shelby, N.C.: Hallelujah Acres. 2002.

Malkmus, George H. *God's Way to Ultimate Health*. Shelby, N.C.: Hallelujah Acres Publishing, 13th Printing, 1999.

Malkmus, George. *The Hallelujah Diet*. Shippensburg, PA: Destiny Image Publishers, Inc. 2006.

Malkmus, George. *Why Christians Get Sick*. Shippensburg, PA: Treasure House, 2000.

Malkmus, George. *You Don't Have to Be Sick!* Shelby, N.C.: Hallelujah Acres Publishing, 1999.

Malkmus, Rhonda. *Recipes for Life...From God's Garden*. Shelby, N.C.: Hallelujah Acres Publishing, 7th Printing, 2001.

McDougall, John. *McDougall's Medicine; Fighting the Big Fat Lies with Fad Free Truth*. 3 DVD Set. Santa Rosa, CA.: John & Mary McDougall, 2004.

Mendelsohn, Robert S. *How to Raise a Health Child...In Spite of Your Doctor*. New York: Ballantine Books, 1984.

Mendelsohn, Robert S. *Confessions of a Medical Heretic*. Chicago: Contemporary Books. 1979.

Oski, Frank A. *Don't Drink Your Milk!* Brushton, NY: Teach Services, Inc., 1996.

Polk, Marilyn. *Hallelujah! Simple Weekly Meal Plans,* Shelby, N.C.:
Hallelujah Acres Publishing, 2005.

Robbins, Joel. *Juicing For Health.* R.W. Tulsa, OK: Graybill &
Company, 2001.

Robbins, Joel. *Pregnancy, Childbirth & Children's Diets.* Tulsa,
OK: R.W. Graybill & Company, 2000.

Robbins, John. *The Food Revolution.* Berkeley, CA: Conari Press, 2001.

Rogers, Adrian, *Back to the Basics.* Atlanta, GA: Walk Through the Bible
Ministries, 1995.

Walker, N. W. *Fresh Vegetable and Fruit Juices.* Prescott, AZ:
Norwalk Press, 1978.

The New York Public Library Writer's Guide to Style and Usage. 1st ed., "A
Stonesong Press Book". New York, NY: Harper Collins Publishers, Inc.,
1994.

Wildmon, Donald E. *Nuggets of Gold.* Tupelo, MS: American Family
Association, p. 70, 1970.